Children at Their Best

by the same author

Baby Shiatsu
Gentle Touch to Help your Baby Thrive
Karin Kalbantner-Wernicke and Tina Haase
Foreword by Dr. Steffen Fischer
Illustrated by Monika Werneke
ISBN 978 1 84819 104 4
eISBN 978 0 85701 086 5

of related interest

Shōnishin
The Art of Non-Invasive Paediatric Acupuncture
Thomas Wernicke
ISBN 978 1 84819 160 0
eISBN 978 0 85701 117 6

Principles of Chinese Medicine
What it is, how it works, and what it can do for you
2nd edition
Angela Hicks
ISBN 978 1 84819 130 3
eISBN 978 0 85701 107 7
Part of the Discovering Holistic Health series

Six Healing Sounds with Lisa and Ted
Qigong for Children
Lisa Spillane
ISBN 978 1 84819 051 1
eISBN 978 0 85701 031 5

The Chinese Book of Animal Powers
Chungliang Al Huang
ISBN 978 1 84819 066 5
eISBN 978 0 85701 037 7

Children at Their Best

Understanding and Using the Five Elements
to Develop Children's Full Potential for
Parents, Teachers, and Therapists

Karin Kalbantner-Wernicke
and Bettye Jo Wray-Fears
With Thomas Wernicke

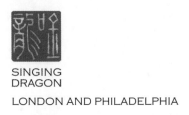

SINGING
DRAGON
LONDON AND PHILADELPHIA

First published in 2014
by Singing Dragon
an imprint of Jessica Kingsley Publishers
73 Collier Street
London N1 9BE, UK
and
400 Market Street, Suite 400
Philadelphia, PA 19106, USA

www.singingdragon.com

Copyright © Karin Kalbantner-Wernicke and Bettye Jo Wray-Fears 2014
Translation copyright © Anne Oppenheimer 2014
Meridian illustrations copyright © aceki e.V. 2014
Photographs copyright © Thomas Wernicke 2014

Library of Congress Cataloging in Publication Data
Kalbantner-Wernicke, Karin, 1956-
  Children at their best : understanding and using the five elements to develop children's full potential
for parents, teachers and therapists / Karin Kalbantner-Wernicke and Bettye Jo Wray-
Fears.
      pages cm.
  Includes bibliographical references and index.
  ISBN 978-1-84819-118-1 (alk. paper)
  1. Child development. 2. Developmental disabilities. 3. Five agents (Chinese philosophy) 4. Child
psychology. 5. Alternative medicine. I. Wray-Fears, Bettye Jo. II. Title.
  RJ131.K35 2014
  618.92--dc23
                            2013048144

British Library Cataloguing in Publication Data
A CIP catalogue record for this book is available from the British Library

ISBN 978 1 84819 118 1
eISBN 978 0 85701 093 3

Printed and bound in Great Britain by Bell & Bain Ltd, Glasgow

Contents

Introduction

Sharing Our Path in Working with the Five Elements in Child Development

What makes this book on child development different? What makes a reader want to find out about an Eastern view integrated with our Western perspective on how children grow? We came to this integration when searching to find ways to offer children greater possibilities to be seen and supported in their development. Since 1990, we have been exploring the overlap of these approaches. As we incorporated and integrated both perspectives into our practice, a broader, more holistic map arose that revealed how the integration of Eastern and Western views can offer support for each stage of life. Today, that larger picture incorporates our growth from infancy, via toddlerhood, childhood, adolescence, and adulthood, through to old age.

This book provides an introduction to this view. We started this exploration by interweaving the Eastern concept of the traditional Five Elements with our knowledge of child development. Since we belong to a Western culture, much of this book reveals how the Eastern view is actually a global view that allows us to return to a macrocosmic and integrated view of life. We invite the reader to explore these complementary, overlapping lenses and thereby find ways to integrate today's modern perspectives with this ancient wisdom that can bring a more holistic approach to supporting our growing children in the world today.

The Five Elements describe something that is innate in all human beings, regardless of language, culture, or where one lives. They represent a cycle in life on many levels. One level is based on the movement, influence, and cycle of the five seasons of our earth—one more than the four seasons we know of in the West. The Five Elements are a system that is analogous to the movement and flow we know to be true in our own bodies and in nature. In Eastern cultures, the Five Elements are recognized as the ancient and archetypal rhythms of life that guide every level of development in nature—plants, animals, and humans. From birth and growth, to reproduction, maturation, aging, and death, particular experiences are shared by all human beings who live a full life.

Before our time of green houses, genetically modified foods, and intensive food production to meet the massive demands of global markets, those who farmed the land knew more certainly the way their lives were intimately linked and affected by the seasons of the year. Connection to the way each season has a different function, level of activity, and outcome to support life was more integrated in our behaviors and survival routines year after year. This experience is lost to many of us in the modern world, with our rapidly expanding technology, crowded population centers, demand for instant results, and scientific developments that defy the laws of nature and the seasons.

As therapists working with children and raising children of our own, we have seen the effects of disconnection from the innate cycles and rhythm of nature and the ways our education, medicine, and parenting have also been skewed. Children today are growing up in a world that is vastly different from the one we knew at their age. And each generation will face new challenges as science and nature diverge more and more.

This book attempts to revive the perspective of the simplicity of the human cycle of birth to death and its inseparable connection to the earth upon which we are raised. It integrates our Western knowledge of the body and the development of the nervous system of our emotional and cognitive capacities with the Eastern view that is analogous to the continuous cycle of the earth's seasons from year to year.

We hope to offer you, and the children you support, a view of life and development that is more holistic and grounded in the realities of life and its cycles, and to provide you with tools and experience in the Five Elements that will bring back the innate rhythm and flow into your lives. The more children are allowed to flow with their innate cycle, the more possibilities there are for them to develop in healthy and whole ways to support their own direction and calling in life.

Traditional Five Element Theory: Connecting Humans with a Natural Rhythm of Life

What are the Five Elements?

For more than 5000 years, Chinese and Japanese medicine have observed the flow of life, from beginning to end, as a cycle. This continuous cycle has five distinct phases that are called the Phases of Change or the Five Elements. The Elements have individual characteristics that are analogous to and connected with nature and the changing seasons of our planet. Like the seasons, each Element cannot exist without the others and is part of a natural flow that affects all of the seasons that follow. The human body, mental faculty, and spirit are not separate from this cycle and are seen as one in the whole dynamic process of life and death. The Five Elements describe the interrelatedness of all things and show how the body, emotions, the mental capacity of the mind, and the spiritual nature of humankind are part of the natural ebb and flow of the earth and the environment.

Truly, *everything* can be understood using the Five Element theory, which reflects the foundational Chinese belief that the only constant in life is change, and that everything we see and can name is part of the movement of this change. This movement of change is described by the cycle of the earth's seasons. Nature itself expresses the rhythm of life and the transformation of all things, animate and inanimate. Each season dictates the unfolding abundance of the next. The cycle is continuous, ever rebalancing and harmonizing, so that life can exist.

The ancient Chinese theory uses five seasons as opposed to the Western four, giving an additional season that honors the transition of all things into the next phase or season in life. The seasons and corresponding elements are Spring–Wood, Summer–Fire, Indian Summer–Earth, Autumn–Metal, and Winter–Water. The Elements flow and follow the same order of the seasons. The diagram and brief descriptions below reveal some of the characteristics that can be related to our human functions in development and daily activities in life.

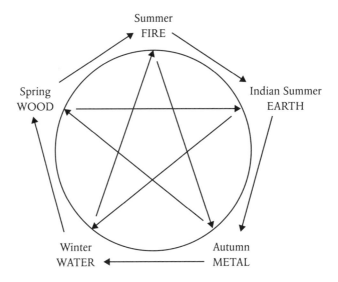

The five seasons and corresponding elements

- *Wood:* Springtime; birth; growth; expansion in all directions, like the seed of an oak tree taking root and sprouting up and down and out from the earth; need for open areas and movement for growth; creativity and planning.

- *Fire:* Summertime; maturation; pollination; reproduction; communication and interrelating of all of nature for balance, like the busy bees pollinating the flowers from tree to tree, and plant to plant, allowing the flowers, fruits, and seeds to be created; warmth and joyful activity.

- *Earth:* Indian Summer; ripening, collecting, storing; digesting and bringing the harvest of life to perfect fruition; nourishment; distributing the harvest to all; the common ground that all the Elements move from; solid and grounded, the center.

- *Metal:* Autumn; harvest time and preparation for the winter; reflection, contemplation, inspiration; letting go of what is no longer needed, like autumn leaves falling from the trees; keeping that which is precious to sustain life-like ores, gems, and metals; discernment and sharpness to cut through what is no longer needed and create boundaries; sense of time with reminder winter is coming next.

- *Water:* Winter; hibernation and rejuvenation of all aspects of life; appearance of stillness and great power; steadfastness; rest and relaxation; conservation of energy; appearance of death and readiness for rebirth.

This summary provides a general description of the qualities of the Elements and their connection to the seasons. The Elements are used to observe every aspect of life, from the developmental stages of a lifetime, to the creation of a company, home, relationship, or simple project. *Everything* is seen to be part of this cycle and have the capacity for balance. When each of the Five Elements are expressed and allowed to mature and transform, then all of the stages and activities in life can find balance.

The Evolution of Five Element Theory and Child Development Work

We first experienced the qualities of the Five Elements with our patients in various settings, ranging from Shiatsu clinics and schools to private allopathic medical practices. Karin Kalbantner-Wernicke and her husband Thomas worked directly with the correlation between the nature of child development and the Five Element view in 1991 when they introduced a children's play therapy called "Spiel-Räume," which means "Room to Play." It was the first approach that directly overlapped Western physical therapy models and tools with the flow of the Five Elements. Originally a physical therapist, Karin was introduced to the Five Elements when she moved to Japan for several years, studying the Japanese medical approach to health while receiving her Shiatsu training in Tokyo.

Here, the roots for the work that started in Germany were planted in the creation of the Institut für Shiatsu in 1981, where the application of the Eastern modality for health and wellbeing was taught and practiced by Karin. It was through the institute that she met Bettye Jo Wray-Fears as one of her early students. Each contributed to the unfolding and articulation of the child development theory and practice offered in this book. Karin and Thomas's continued studies, inquiry, and experimentation have led to an even more comprehensive perspective on how the Eastern energetic map overlaps and offers a broad, practical view that complements our Western knowledge of human development from birth to death.

In our first book, *Spiel-Räume: Die Fünf Elemente im Leben von Kindern* (*Room to Play: The Five Elements in the Lives of Children*), an additional author also contributed to the foundation of the early exploration of working with children and the Five Elements, Susanne Löhner-Jokisch. In that text, we introduced the early theory of the Five Elements to integrate not only the physical issues of sensory development the children were experiencing but also the emotional and mental development that seemed to go hand in hand. Karin offered the experiential background and evidence for this work from her specialized children's play therapy program, Spiel-Räume (Room to Play), which integrated Western physical therapy with traditional Five Element theory. Bettye Jo supported the integration of these two disciplines, incorporating her Western psychological background and her in-depth knowledge of the Five Elements gained from training in the United States. Susanne offered further insight, examples, and exercises from her experience with kindergarten classes, and Thomas contributed in-depth knowledge and evidence from the Western–Eastern medical integration in his clinic specializing in child development. Further information on the authors' backgrounds may be found at the end of the book.

Our particular interest is to demonstrate the power and natural effectiveness that the Five Elements can bring to your interactions with children, whether as parents, families, teachers, mentors, or therapists. This book offers a rich history of more than 20 years' experience collected personally from working with the Five Elements in our practices. The integration of our Western approaches with Five Element theory gave us room to see human development and children's behavior in a new way. For therapists, parents, teachers, and mentors, it is a guide to creating supportive environments for the children we work with. For children, the Five Elements offer new freedom for balanced growth and personal expression of what is moving inside them.

We invite you to stop right now for a moment and reflect on the children you live or work with. If you think about your experience of watching children play, you can probably recognize that most like to run and tumble, create imaginary games, build castles together, and sing. We have also observed through our work ranges of normal progression in children, in their interest and ability to participate in group activities from early preschool ages to elementary school years. Those children who have found "normal" pathways to express the stimulation of activity around them interact in a playground or group setting such as a classroom with ease and enjoyment. They laugh, jump, climb, and play happily with one another.

If you are reading this book, however, you have probably also noticed first-hand that this natural progression is missing for many children. Equally noticeable are those who appear withdrawn or over-cautious, or those who lack a sense of boundaries with respect to others or their own personal safety. These children are often unhappy, or they may be the instigators of problems for others in the group.

One of the first questions we asked in the early development of the Five Element perspective was: "Are these children choosing to act this way, or is this the only behavior they are capable of at this time?" A typical Western approach would overlook difficult behavior in early childhood development, and expect that the child would outgrow their difficulties. Unfortunately, this doesn't happen for many children. How do we explain, then, those children whose behavior and maturity does not match the "average" expectations for their age? How do we explain and guide those who do not grow and mature at an "acceptable pace" in their behavioral, physical, and mental development?

From the perspective of the Five Elements, it was clear that in order to reveal new possibilities for understanding and guiding children's development we needed to explore the latter part of the question. In time, our inquiry and our question expanded to include not only "Is this the only behavior this child is capable of at this time?" but also "*What* is this child expressing at this time, and why isn't he or she capable of more?" After years of working with children labeled "challenged" by our Western educational and medical models, we found this inquiry could be answered more fruitfully using the understanding of the Five Elements. The Five Elements provided another framework to observe, explain, connect, and support the integration of Western concepts that continued to expand our child development work.

Each time we came together to discuss our child development work, our clients, and our own therapeutic practices and lives, it became apparent that the original "Spiel-Räume" intentions extended well beyond the therapy room. The work was opening the natural flow of the Five Elements in our lives, the lives of our clients, and even their extended family members. We were deeply moved that this ancient model described and awakened something already present within our clients and ourselves—some innate, subtle force that links all races, all cultures, and, indeed, all humanity together.

This was the process that inspired the first book in Germany, which continues to be dedicated to all the children, families, and clients who walked that journey of awakening with us. The inspiration derived from this work has been a gift in our lives. With our continued growth and experience, we found ourselves asking a very important question: "What do we want from this work?" Our answers came as spontaneously as the question:

- We want children to be seen and understood in a different light—one that supports their unique gifts, challenges, and potential.

- We want to empower those courageous adults who take on the responsibility to teach, counsel, and care for our children with a deeper understanding of human development.

- We want children's lives to be touched in a way that gives them room to grow and express all the aspects of the Five Elements in their own balanced, unique way.

- We want to create a guide for adults so they can discover and integrate simple, effective techniques in their environment and practices that will offer balanced expressions of the Five Elements and support the children they are working with.

- We want to offer examples from our experience so that the reader can relate to and be inspired by the children they work with and their struggles in life.

- We want others to feel stirred and touched by something familiar in this work—something that is innate and brings a familiar sensation of a natural rhythm and balance that they already know and can share with others.

We want to make it clear that the underlying concepts of this book are not new, nor were they discovered by us. In the context of our own lives and professional practices, we have incorporated a combination of Eastern and Western approaches that supports the integration, roundedness, and multiplicity of child development. The Five Elements provide a common ground that holds true for all expressions of life.

We hope that sharing the work in the book will give you a feeling for the Five Elements and the way they already exist in your life. This book is for children who need to be seen and supported in all their diversity, for parents, teachers, and therapists who are looking for ways to meaningfully support them, and the longing of life itself to find its unique expression and live fully.

Children are our future. Educators, therapists, caretakers, and parents are their doorways. The room we give our children to play and grow will affect the future of the whole world.

PART I

Child Development Theory and the Five Elements

CHAPTER 1

How Do Children Develop?
Overlapping the Western and Eastern Views

We would like to acknowledge Dr. Thomas Wernicke as a contributing writer to this chapter, and co-creator, with Karin Kalbantner-Wernicke, of the East–West model of energetic development of children that this book presents. His expertise in Western and Eastern medicine with children in his clinic has not only allowed the picture of how children come into their bodies energetically and physically to become clear, but also has supported this view through the evidence of healing with many infants, babies, and children in Germany.

Children are full of curiosity and thirsty for action. Each day they learn more about themselves and their surroundings. They develop individually through this learning process, and the progression is very similar from child to child. Development occurs naturally and follows a pattern that has both individual and universal characteristics. Children develop at different speeds, constantly making smaller or larger strides.

If you are a parent, you may remember talking to others with children and comparing your three-month-old babies. One was larger and stronger, another quite dainty ("the little lady"), another one fidgety ("My husband was like that when he was little!"), and another mostly slept. Remember what happened in playgroups? Did your child pile up blocks two and three high like the others— fortunately!—or did something seem different somehow ("He/she was so tensed up…")?

Through such comparisons with other children the same age, a difference in development can sometimes prompt uncertainty in parents, since many parents do not know how to evaluate their own observations. They ask themselves if their child's development still falls within the "norm," or whether it is delayed or unbalanced. Sometimes parents are falsely reassured by relatives and friends in these situations, or they are needlessly unsettled by labels that suggest the child is not developing in the natural developmental stages.

If you work with children in any capacity, or simply have the opportunity to observe your children playing with a large variety of playmates, then you know that some children end up in a sort of dead-end street. Some develop above-average skills in one area, while showing avoidance behavior in others. You may also have observed hypersensitive children who become overwhelmed by stimulus from the environment and react in maladaptive ways because they don't know how to explain their perceptions of their surroundings. There are also children who become overtaxed because particular skills and tasks are expected of them too soon. These and other children often struggle with an inability to progress in their development, simultaneously encountering an education system that is not given the room or tools to work with them.

The boundaries between normal and delayed development are difficult to define, partly because there are many different types of senses developing at different rates at the same time in each child, and many different opinions about what a child should be capable of at different ages. Newer approaches in child development are now acknowledging the importance of bonding, attachment, and physical movement as major foundations for healthy child development. At the same time, the education system in the US is struggling to make financial decisions, with some areas of the country removing physical education from the school day, and others even removing lunch periods. Deprivation of contact and face-to-face relating in an increasingly technological world of cell phones and computers is also a factor that will need to be explored in the future as we look at the evolution of children in the world. These and the multiple factors of Western diagnoses, such as attention deficit disorders, sensory sensitivities, autistic spectrum disorders and defiant disorders, continue to add to the list of ways traditional Western medicine approaches and treats children who struggle.

From the Five Element perspective, it is important that developmental and learning delays are not viewed as an illness in a child. Rather, they are part of a whole process, created by a disharmony in the child's overall internal and/or external environment during development. To understand this premise, we need to look at a summary of the overlapping Eastern and Western views of child development. We have chosen to focus more on the Eastern concepts and present the new material that this book is based on, rather than give in-depth detail of the Western terms that most parents, educators, therapists, and mentors already have access to.

Overlapping East and West in Child Development

Western medicine observes child development from many different perspectives. Two primary development theories we will focus on with the energetic development in this section will be sensory development and motor development. Before we begin to overlap these two approaches, however, we want to point out that the term "energetic development" is misleading in that it is often viewed as something that is intangible.

The word "energy" is loosely used in the West to refer to everything from our individual stamina and feeling to scientific facts about energy and what makes our electronic and transportation world function. Even though the West uses a concept of energy transformation daily when calculating the calories in the food we eat, the physical functions and systems of the human body are rarely described in terms of an energetic transformation. Modern medicine and quantum physics are researching daily how our bodies interact with the environment and how our minds affect our biological functions. The term is often used even more loosely in discussions between doctors and patients who describe their overall "energy level" with symptoms of fatigue or daily-life activity levels.

So the concept of energy is not completely foreign to our Western minds when we enter the topic of Eastern medicine and energy. This book will talk about energy from a more micro- and macrocosmic perspective which is used in the Eastern medical approach as an integral understanding of how energy supports the functions of the body.

Energy is called *Ki* in Japanese; when asking "How are you?" in Japanese, this concept is included in the phrase "O gen*ki* desu ka?" This phrase alone shows how the concept of energy is an integral part of the Japanese view of health and the body—the Eastern medical approach does not separate energy from daily health. It considers the function of energy in the body to be as important as the blood that flows through the veins to support all the organs and life-sustaining systems.

The Eastern medical model also applies this concept of lack of separation of energy from the physical functions of the body to the developmental stages of children. When we talk about a child learning to stand up, for example, from the developmental perspective of the Five Element approach, we see that there are "energetic" structures that influence the development of muscles, coordination, and brain development, which are part of the process of the body's physical development. In the Eastern medical approach, the view is that the energy/*Ki* moves first in the body and needs the physical movement of the body to ground the pattern of movement for the energetic pathways. This gives the *Ki* awareness or memory to continue to move through the body and support physical movement and development. The *Ki* is the precursor to the developmental movements a child makes, and continues to be the initiator of all movement even after the muscles and nervous system have learned the energetic path and physical pattern of movement. They are dependent on each other to function.

Every physical activity the body is involved in is influenced by and intermingled with a *Ki* activity. This basic premise alone is what we ask readers to open their minds to and experiment with in the exercises and examples that are offered.

Principles of Child Development

When we talk about the development of children and overlapping our lenses of Eastern and Western dialogue, we will talk about children developing on three different levels. The three principles of development are presented individually, although all are entirely

dependent on each other and develop at the same time. Below is a
brief description of how these systems apply to a growing child:

1. *Motor development* is the way we learn to crawl, to stand
   upright, and to move. Motor development is further broken
   down into two levels known as gross and fine motor skills.
   Gross motor skills are the ability to make large movements—
   such as running, jumping, and climbing. Fine motor skills
   are the ability to make small, more detailed movements—for
   example, holding a cup or a spoon, stacking blocks on top of
   one another, and, eventually, writing.

2. *Sensory development* is the development of the senses we have
   to perceive ourselves and the world around us—for example,
   seeing, hearing, tasting, smelling, and touching. Our ability to
   differentiate textures, colors, objects, sounds, smells, and tastes
   is dependent on our sensory development. Some children
   are born over-sensitive (hyper) or under-sensitive (hypo) in
   different senses, which can make it difficult for these children
   to focus and participate in group activities with others.

3. *Energetic development* refers to the overall development of a
   child with an understanding of the interdependent nature
   of the biological, motor, sensory, cognitive, emotional, and
   energetic developing systems that are influenced by the total
   environment in which a child grows up and interacts. The
   energetic model of development combines knowledge of
   modern neuroscience, and developmental physiology with
   the knowledge and experience of traditional Eastern and
   Japanese medicine. It is based on the Eastern principle that
   everything consists of energy and uses the Eastern energetic
   model of the body with stages of development that occur
   from birth to adult. In the energetic developmental model,
   the human being has the possibility to continue developing
   throughout a lifetime.

Motor Development

It is a miracle that we can stand, walk, and even run given how
undeveloped we are as newborns. The stages of motor development

to be completed from infancy to independent movement are immense. Each minor level of motor development is dependent on the preceding one, and each lays the foundation for much more than just the physical movements of the body.

We can see this by looking at a primary movement of a six-month-old baby and examining the sequence of motor development. What does a baby of this age do when she is lying on her stomach and wants to lift her head to see something? Typically, she is able to move her arms out in front of her and then lean her weight into her hands and thighs as she pushes her head up, lifting herself off her elbows and upper torso so that she can turn her head from side to side or look up. But what if the motor development of her arms was delayed in some way and she didn't know how to use her arms—how then would she manage this movement?

Try it yourself! Lie on your stomach. Keep your arms at your side or very close to the body and try lifting your head to see around the room. You have to pull your head back into your neck, arch the back, and push your weight into your pelvis while your legs strain and your knees lift from the floor. As adults, we can all find a way to do this movement with more or less effort.

For a child, however, if the "armless" way described above was the only way to raise the head and see something in the room, because of a developmental delay or lack of room for discovery, then a forced pattern of movement would be created and used exclusively. Through constant repetition of such a pattern, the brain learns and is "imprinted." Since lifting the head is one of the first developmental movements a child must learn, a child faced with a delayed development of the arms may now begin all other new movements from this one imprinted pattern. Even if it takes more energy and strength to move from this awkward imprint, the brain has not had the chance to learn another way. The result is the development of what is called "a pathological movement pattern." Pathological movement patterns are created when there is a discrepancy between what a child is capable of doing and what a child wants to do.

To broaden this idea, let's return to the original example of the delayed development of the six-month-old baby above. This time, get a few friends to try lifting their heads while lying on their stomachs without the use of their arms. What do you notice now? Most likely, you will see some differences in the way each person is able to follow through with this limited movement—some may not be able to do it at all!

This happens because we all develop our own particular patterns of movements. These patterns develop as our brain becomes imprinted from repetition. We repeated the movements our body was developmentally capable of and within the space our environment allowed. There really is no right or wrong way to do a given movement. Only the order of development is of consequence. The variety of ways in which the adults were able to perform the no-arms movement demonstrates this concept.

Our brain has the capacity to perform the same activity in many different ways; this is an important ability of the human brain that we should recognize. How is this possible? Research shows that this capacity for variety begins with movements very early on in our development. During the seventh week of pregnancy, movement of a developing child can be observed. This is a key time for the beginning development of the initial movement patterns that will lead to multiple avenues and choices later in adult life. Let's have a look at a very basic description of the nervous system and the ways in which it develops in a fetus.

The entire nervous system is comprised of the brain and its five basic components—the two cerebral hemispheres, brain stem, spinal cord, and smaller cerebellum—and numerous nerves that branch out through the whole body. Nerve cells are called neurons, which we will simplify into two categories: sensory neurons and motor neurons. Sensory neurons send information from the body to the brain, and motor neurons send information from the brain to the organs and muscles of the body.

The movement of the fetus stimulates the development of the brain as sensory neuron after sensory neuron forms infinite connections (synapses) and pathways, from the stimulus to the brain. Control centers are established as a result of the linking nerve synapses and pathways, and the brain responds by sending responses back to the organs and muscles through the motor neurons. In the first months of life, brain development is entirely dependent on the movement of the fetus so that countless control centers and neural pathways can be created. And, in precisely the same way, everything we learn later after birth will continue the development of our brain.

We have billions of neuron cells just waiting to learn and connect stimuli from the outer world into new movements or already existing imprinted patterns of movement. To know more alternative movements means to have freedom of choice and, as a result, to have a greater ability to act in many situations in life.

To apply this knowledge to our children means we should nurture and encourage different forms of movement. Giving many choices and experiences broadens the base for children to develop on all levels.

The box below gives information about the chronological order of movement patterns as a child develops—milestones of motor development. These represent average ages.

When we follow the motor development of a child during the first two years of life in the box above, it becomes clear that restrictions of movement affect more than just physical development. Can you imagine what would happen if a child had nothing in her environment to stimulate eye movement in the first three months of life, or if, out of fear, her space was limited so that she was not allowed to move and turn to the side, front, or back? Attempts to move and explore one's environment are some of a child's first "planning" strategies. Anyone who has witnessed a child growing has experienced a child's frustrated cry or sounds when she can't get to an object, person, or activity she desires.

Limited exploration of movement and restricted motor development play a very important role in the later psychological and emotional stages of life. For this reason, the term "restricted freedom of movement" should be understood to mean also a restriction of our freedom to think, act, and plan. For balanced development, every child needs her own room to play, an environment that enables her to move and explore with the least amount of limitation.

Milestones of motor development

Birth. The newborn stretches, and moves its bottom and its limbs.

First month. In the first month, an infant can briefly raise and turn her head while lying on her stomach. The arms remain close to the body and the hands form loose fists.

Second month. Lying on the stomach, an infant can briefly hold her head up and follow movements to the right and left. The infant can support her body on her forearms and also suck her thumb or the backs of her hands.

Third month. In the third month, an infant can hold her head in a middle position while lying on her back, and begins to bring the hands together at the midline and sides of the feet touching together. Hand to hand, and foot to foot, the infant gets more connected to the self. When on the stomach, the body is supported on the forearms and the infant can turn her head freely.

Fourth month. On her back, the baby continues to explore the hand-to-hand and foot-to-foot experience. On her stomach, the baby uses her forearms to raise her upper body and head. She can grasp as intended and can hold objects in her hands.

Fifth month. On her stomach, the baby can now support herself briefly with outstretched arms, or on only one elbow and forearm, while the free hand seeks to grasp things. When on her back, the baby can sometimes roll onto the stomach. Objects can be transferred from one hand to the other.

Sixth month. At six months, we have the hand-to-foot contact stage. A child can hold the feet playfully with the hands. Now the baby begins to turn on either side, but prefers one side. Holding tight with the hands, she can pull herself up into a sitting position. She has good head control, which is a prerequisite for discovering her surroundings. In addition, flat, tong-like grasping (with the whole hand and opposing thumb) is now possible.

Seventh month. In the seventh month, the baby can raise her head while lying on one side. Rolling is now fully developed and the baby begins to wriggle, but this mostly ends up as sliding backwards. The baby still favors the tong-like grip but smaller objects can be grasped with thumb and bent forefinger (pincer-grip).

Eighth month. Many but not all babies can balance on the hands and knees (the four-leg position). She gradually begins pulling herself into an upright position on the knees by herself while being supported by furniture or others. She explores her surroundings and makes continued efforts to reach something in the room. The pincer-grip is favored. There is great interest in details and small objects, and the baby points with the forefinger at tiny crumbs and wants to pick them up. This stage can be called the "crumb stage."

From this point onwards, further development varies significantly according to the individual child, but we would nonetheless like to give several clues.

Ninth month. Lying on the stomach or back is now used only for sleeping. From her side, the baby will now sit up, sit still for a moment, and then begin to pull herself up to stand. She begins to crawl.

Tenth month. The tenth month is the transitional stage between the horizontal and a still unstable vertical: the child holds on to objects to pull herself up and begins to move sideways along the edges of furniture. She can hold a spoon but must still be fed.

Eleventh month. Now she sits up by herself and is balanced while sitting. She tries to stand up unaided. All means of grasping are available.

Twelfth month. She crawls everywhere and can take a few free steps.

Fifteenth month. Walking without any help or support for several meters is possible, with the sense of balance not yet fully imprinted, and she can go into a crouched position.

Eighteenth month. She stands without assistance from furniture or others, can change direction while walking without falling, clambers up on to couches, and goes up the stairs while holding on to something.

Twenty-fourth month. When the child is supported, she can hop on two feet.

The progress of motor development presented here occurs at genetically programmed stages without human intervention. The order and the qualitative progression of each child can vary.

Sensory Development

Seeing, hearing, touching, tasting, and smelling are the five senses we rely on every day of our lives to understand and communicate with our surroundings. Like the influence of motor development on the neural development of the body and brain, these primary senses play just as large a role in the development of the nervous system. Every movement creates a sensory perception for the body, and every sensory perception promotes a movement. Before a child learns to move, he must be able to feel. For this, he needs doors to the exterior world. The senses are those doorways because they give the body the ability to receive sensory information.

If you recall the basic description of the development of the nervous system in the previous section, it stated that the sensory neurons transmit information from the body to the brain. Sensory neurons receive their stimulus from sensory receptors that receive information from the environment through vibrations, pressure, movement, light, texture, smells, tastes, and sounds. The sensory receptors are the openings through which a child gains information about his body and his environment.

The progression of sensory development is not as easily defined as the progression of motor development. This is because observation of sensory activity (sensations felt by the fetus) is only possible (detectable) when there is some kind of motor response, movement, or physical reaction in the developing child.

Let's look at a brief summary of what we know about the beginnings of sensory development in a child. The interaction between motor activity and sensory activity begins in the womb. Around the second month of gestation, the neurons begin to multiply and spread out to the periphery of the developing body. As soon as these basic neural cells are created, they begin performing their function of sensing, sending sensory input in and out of the developing brain, and back out to the appropriate developing organs, muscles, tendons, and tissues. All of the mother's movements offer stimulus for the developing neural system, and all of the infant's motor and developmental organ responses as well.

The process of the interplay between sensory and motor development occurs like this: the developing child initially receives information through contact with the amniotic fluid. It feels the pressure of the liquid against the skin and responds with movements against the pressure. This gives a variety of information and gentle stimulus to the developing muscles, tendons, joints, and ligaments. The brain receives each stimulus and more neural pathways are created. Each time the sensory neurons of the fetus "feel," a sensory stimulus occurs. The response to each sensory stimulus is a movement or motor response. Sensory development and motor development become inseparable, and the development of the brain is dependent on the interplay between them.

This happens around the clock through the interaction of the mother and her developing child. The mother's own blood supplies the nutrition, and her movements, rhythmic heartbeat, and breathing pattern offer stimulation to the fetus. Just as importantly, stimulation also comes from the developing child's movements in response to its *in utero* experience and outer environment. As the fetus continues to grow, it is able to touch the uterine wall itself with its arms, hands, legs, and feet. It responds to sound from the mother's surroundings: music, familial voices, and sudden loud noises. Motor responses to bright lights and colors have been observed—even when the eyelids of the fetus are closed. Heart rate differences and movements have been detected in the fetus when the mother has contact with others or the belly is massaged or stroked.

Like motor development, the stages of sensory development that occur during pregnancy lay the foundation for further sensory development in infancy and early childhood. An infant is born with all five senses and also a sense of gravity and movement. The level of development at birth is a very basic foundation. From the moment the child is born, the brain continues to develop and find ways to interpret and respond to the new surroundings and environment in the same way it did *in utero*. The environmental and self-sensory stimuli that are experienced constantly by the developing child, in and out of the womb, are essential for the brain to develop—they are the nerve nourishment for the brain.

If we compare the very basic level of senses and motor responses we are born with or develop in the first month to what is available in a two-year-old, it would be hard to deny that the development is profound. By the time a child is two years old, he is capable of running and standing on tiptoe. He can blow a horn or harmonica, has begun to talk a little, and can communicate very well what he wants and does not want to do.

How does this huge leap of development happen? It manifests step by step, one neural synapse after another—a demonstration of the brain's amazing ability to organize stimuli from the environment and turn them into efficient, appropriate responses. The steps to this process are so intricate and unique to each child that science does not yet know all of the stages that take place in our neurological development.

We can see that sensory development begins very early, that there is some kind of chronological order of development achieved by certain ages, and that it is a building-block type of process. The sense of touch is one of the primary senses for the foundation of many developments in life. In the infant's life, the hands are like the mouth—carriers of information, through which he experiences his world. Through grasping, an infant learns about the world. When we forbid our child to grasp things, we close off the possibility for him to learn about his surroundings. For this reason, we should give our children every chance to feel the world through their principal sense organ, the skin. This allows them to develop not only the sense of physical textures in the world but also information about themselves, their fellow human beings, and their environment.

Through motor development, children learn to move their hands and all the parts of their bodies. Through sensory development, the hands become organs of perception and learn how to grasp different objects. As children advance in the combinations of motor and sensory development in the hands, we can observe how the hands become a means of communication.

Gesture comes into play, used alone at first, then later as an accompaniment to speech. Children support their speech through lively gesticulations, and this form of communication, culturally defined through upbringing, will be restricted to a greater or lesser degree.

These are only a few examples of how early sensory and motor development support later major areas of development in our life. When we observe the early struggles that children have in their development and compare it to our own adult inadequacies, we can't help but question how early motor and sensory development affects many of our behaviors and abilities in adulthood. Before we go any further in that exploration, however, it is important to consider another stage of development that sets the scene for our whole approach—energetic development.

Energetic Development

This book is based on how the Five Elements affect and can be worked with in child development. Before going into details about the theory of the Five Elements, however, it's important to understand what energetic development is and how a child develops into the Five Elements.

As in development in the Western model, the Eastern energetic model has stages that are like building blocks creating the foundation for each other as a child grows and matures. In this overview of energetic development, we outline the basic principles of Eastern medicine and the stages of energetic development that lead to the mature state of being able to develop fully in the Five Elements.

Similar to the way in which a child is born unable to walk and must develop many levels of sensory and motor skills before being able to achieve this integrated physical capacity, so too is a child unable to function in the Five Elements fully until after maturing in the elementary stages and structures of the *Ki* energy present from birth to about five to seven years old. This does not mean that the Five Elements are not considered in the observation of a developing child until five to seven years old. On the contrary, the way the whole environment expresses the Five Elements in a child's life and responds to expressions of the child that belong to the Five Elements is still observed in the same way one would observe how they are supporting a child's environment for learning how to stand and early attempts to walk.

THE FOUNDATION OF ENERGETIC DEVELOPMENT: KI, THE LIFE FORCE

Everything in the universe is made up of a life force or energy. All phenomena in nature, all animate and inanimate objects, are made of, propelled by, and transformed into various forms of the life force. This may seem like a very abstract concept to many of us brought up in the Western world. In actuality, however, the Western scientific approach is based on a similar awareness that operates on the premise that everything in existence is made up of atoms. The air that we breathe, the food that we eat, the ground and chairs that support us—and even our bodies—are made up of these common single particles. They have positive and negative charges, energy, that allows them to combine with each other to transform and create all substances. Atoms are charged particles that are the foundation for all gaseous, aqueous, and solid matter. In Western science, all living things and inanimate objects are understood to share this common element in their basic structure.

Similarly, the Eastern view connects all phenomena in our world through the explanation of a *life force* or energy called *Ki* in Japanese, or *Chi* in Chinese. This *Ki* is the foundation for Eastern traditions of medicine, philosophy, martial arts, and the overall cultural perspective. It is the common substance of all gaseous, aqueous, and solid matter. In the energetic development of a child, *Ki* begins with the constitutional energy that is created by the combination of the mother's and father's energy at the moment of conception. Similar to the DNA and RNA present at conception, so too the life force for the child created at conception has an imprint and propensity to develop certain characteristics and capacities with the right stimulus from the environment as the child develops. As the fetus develops, its *Ki* is further affected by the mother's health and the environment she lives in during the pregnancy.

The *Ki* of a child at birth continues to be stimulated by the environment throughout the child's life and affects the energetic development step by step in the course of the maturation from infancy to old age. The physical elements of air, climate, food, and water are the natural manifestations of *Ki* in the surroundings. The psychological and emotional settings created by the parents and significant others, the physical space, and the way a child is held and encouraged to explore and learn about the world will also enhance or hinder the *Ki* and energetic development.

MERIDIANS: THREE PHASES OF DEVELOPMENT

At the moment of conception, the *Ki* transforms into an energetic field that is like the engine and fuel, all in one, for the fetus. It is the developing child's own energy from this moment on and will act as a buffer and catalyst for integrating all experiences from the environment and surroundings as the child goes through life.

This energy field takes on a form in the body called meridians, or energy pathways. They are the pathways through which the *Ki* moves in the body.

There are 12 primary meridians of the body. Meridians are energy pathways that connect the deeper organs, tissues, and muscles with the outer-most surface level, the skin; and the inner cognitive, emotional, and social developmental stages.

Some features of meridians that are key to understanding this work are:

- Meridians are inner and outer pathways that allow the energy/ *Ki* to flow through the organs and tissues of the body.

- Meridians exist in an incomplete form at birth and are dependent on the sensory and motor development of a child.

- Meridians need movement and stimulation from the body to develop, and the body needs movement from the meridians to develop.

- Meridians are constantly forming in a growing child and are used to understand the way a child is developing their posture, movement, personality, and social behavior patterns.

- Meridians are part of the Five Element system and are used to work with all of the physical, mental, emotional, and stage of life correspondences.

PHASE 1: THE THREE FAMILIES

At the time of birth, the grid of the 12 primary meridians is laid down, but the meridians are not fully differentiated or functioning. Two energetic phases of development must occur within a child before the 12 primary meridians can differentiate fully into their individual functions.

The first phase of development starts right after birth and continues until the child is walking freely. From birth to the point of walking, the grid of the 12 undeveloped meridians is busy developing and differentiating into three clusters called the *Front*, *Back*, and *Lateral Family* systems. These three groups are each made up of four of the primary 12 meridians. The term "Family" was chosen to describe more clearly the close intermeshing functions of the four unfolding meridians in each of the three groups. Each group acts as a family integrating the sensorimotor, psychological, and energetic systems of development, and their names describe the directional themes that the Three Families are developing. This amazing and intricate phase in the first year of the Three Families is the foundation for a child's energetic development (see the *Baby Shiatsu* book in the Resources section for a full explanation).

In this first developmental phase, the course is set for our later movement through life, and likewise the lenses through which we will view the world. This first year is where the foundation is being laid for the subsequent energetic development of the Five Elements. So each of the Three Families has its own themes in terms of life and development. These themes are part of the pre-cognitive and early cognitive structures that help to support how our inner attitudes will develop and change in our lives. Below is a brief description of the themes of the Three Families, how they are connected to the differentiated meridians later in life, and how they are connected to the themes for the Five Elements later in life.

The Front Family

The Front Family develops in the first year, and later, in the third phase of meridian development, will become the Stomach, Spleen, Large Intestine, and Lung meridians. The Front Family lays the foundation for the Earth and Metal Elements later in life.

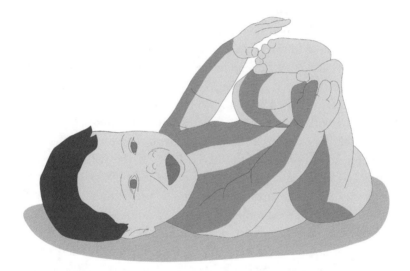

Significance for Earth and Metal Elements: If the qualities of the Front Family can unfold in a child, it means that in later life he will be capable of engaging with new situations and being open with other people. In relation to everyday life at school, it means that he is in a position to form relationships with schoolmates and teachers. In this way, the foundation is laid for success in learning, which ultimately is based on good relationships. If children are open and interested in the new content of what they are taught, and engage with it, this too is a result of the ability to form relationships that they acquired early in life.

The ability to make contact with people involves being able to turn towards them and to make and maintain eye contact. This means being present in oneself and in the space around. Finding and keeping one's own center, independently of what is going on in the environment, and tolerating other points of view (and, when necessary, being able to change one's own view) are also supported by the themes in the realm of the Front Family. Anyone who stands up for their own opinion also risks contradiction and criticism. The ability to handle this and not take it personally also represents someone who has developed strong roots in the Front Family. People who are "thin-skinned" find this very difficult. The organ of the skin (which is related to the Metal Element) and the expressions "to have a thin skin" and "that gets under my skin" can be signs of different sensitivities developed from this family.

For a baby, "getting to grips" with a world that is still strange to her begins with touching, one of a small child's most elementary experiences. She sucks her thumb; her hands touch each other over the chest at the center of the body; later on she will explore her thighs and knees, and finally end up at her feet.

In the time after birth, a baby cannot yet distinguish between "this is me" and "this is somebody else," as the baby lies on his back with various objects appearing in the field of vision. Whether it's the play of shadows on the wall, or the baby's own hand or the mother's hand, the baby can't identify or make associations with what he sees—he simply perceives the stimuli. Only when he finds his center, and further develops the sense of touch that is linked with it, does the baby learn to make the distinction between his own hand and his mother's.

So touch is a sensory system that belongs to the Front Family. By means of touch, the baby, like grown-ups, experiences and comprehends the world. By means of the tactile sense, the baby gets to know his body. He learns "Where do I begin? Where do I end?" and he learns to feel at home in his body. Resting in self, with a sense of his own center, a child can pay attention to the external world and meet it. As the mother and other caretakers respect the responses of a child to the type of touch he needs and wants—allowing the child to have space or holding when he wants it—and respect the child's curiosity to touch objects and textures, the foundation for respect and boundaries for self and others is laid down.

THE BACK FAMILY

The Back Family system will later differentiate into the Bladder, Kidney, Heart, and Small Intestine meridians. The Back Family is, then, the foundation for the Water Element and half of the foundation for the Fire Element (the last two meridians associated with Fire will be part of the Lateral Family).

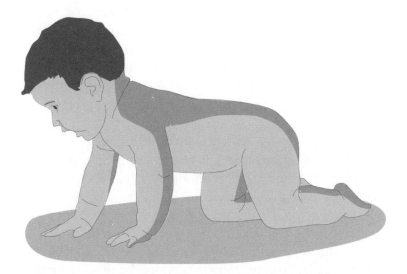

Significance for Water and Fire Elements: The Back Family development will support the development of the Fire Element qualities that deal with a sense of purpose in life and will provide the *Ki* in the Water Element for an internal, external, and physical "upright" capacity in life.

In the first few months of a child's life, experiences of lying on the stomach while being supervised stimulate a child to lift the head and use the developing back muscles to look around in the environment. Examples from the children's clinic in Germany, as well as the work of other physical therapists, doctors, and midwives, have shown that children who have not been offered this opportunity have difficulties in the alignment of the spine and posture which can show up when they get to school. Headaches, difficulty sitting upright in a chair during a school day, becoming easily fatigued, and even speech problems are some of the symptoms observed.

If a school child is constantly occupied with the effort it takes to stay upright on his chair, he can't keep his attention on what he is being taught. A person who is struggling with his posture all the time ultimately has no space in his head for learning.

We have also observed that school-age children with extreme scoliosis or postures with the shoulders hunched forward often have lower self-esteem and more pronounced insecurities, which can lead to giving up prematurely before trying something new in life. "I can't do it anyway!" is often a chronic statement and symbol of a child lacking the "upright stance" needed to meet new challenges and unknowns in life. This "upright stance" is first supported in the development of the Back Family meridian in the first phase of energetic development, and is key to exploring this stage of development in a child as well as difficulties in the later stages of life.

Other signs of this can show with children who demonstrate the feeling that too much is being asked of them, a fear of failure, feeling discouraged, or continual resignation. Often the inward and outward attitude of such a child does not invite communication, another factor that points to looking at possible early disruptions in the development of the Back Family. Language, listening, and the ability to wait your turn are fundamental for good communication. The foundation for the development of speech and language belongs to this family. In particular, children who did not crawl or crawled with fisted hands can be seen to experience difficulties with speech and understanding of math.

In contrast, children who develop a healthy Back Family system are supported later in the Five Elements with an ability to be upright in life, manifesting independence, self-reliance, and an ability to find one's feet in relation to gravity. This leads to increased self-confidence and an ability to evaluate one's own powers. Part of this is being able to recognize when it's necessary to retreat in life. Babies do indeed sense when they should withdraw or need a break, before turning to someone to invite contact again. Babies allowed this experience are supported in developing an inner knowing and allowing of oneself to withdraw for the sake of recovery and rejuvenation in many situations of life.

Confidence that one will find support ("backing") or restraint ("holding back") in life also has early roots in the foundation of the Back Family. "Eight-month anxiety" in infants is one of the first expressions of this: at this stage the infant experiences unfamiliar surroundings and strangers as the loss of a safe and trusted home; children who up until now have approached people they didn't know now hide anxiously behind their mothers. Only once the child has become familiar with the strange person, step by step, will his uncertainty abate. If the child is allowed to gain control of the strange, new world and developing perspective at his own pace, and is encouraged to seek support and safety from his mother whenever he needs it, then he can approach this new world with curiosity and a "broad back," and will move through this uncertain and fearful stage of development, which is called rapprochement in modern psychology.

The Lateral Family

The Lateral Family system will later differentiate into the Gall Bladder, Liver, Pericardium, and Triple Heater meridians. The Lateral Family is, then, the foundation for the Wood Element and half of the foundation for the Fire Element, as the other two meridians associated with Fire are part of the Back Family.

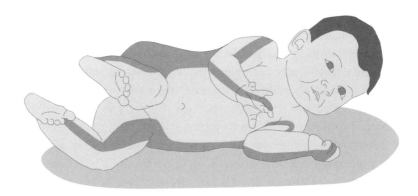

Significance for Wood and Fire Elements: Once the qualities of the Lateral Family have emerged, a capability that has enormous lifelong importance is revealed: that of rotation—one of the most frequent movements in our everyday lives. Rotation facilitates flexibility, which is relevant to all situations in life and is a quality of the Wood Element. Being flexible means being able to negotiate and make compromises—for example, the ability to agree on a project that's based on other people's ideas and, if the general consensus so requires, being able to make changes or adjustments.

Furthermore, for a baby, rotation means the first rolling or turning movements, mastering space, and later balancing along the top of a low wall. This form of movement, which is so important for further development, makes it possible for us to turn towards or away from, or even "turn a cold shoulder." It offers the foundation for facilitating flexibility in all life situations. That is possible only by crossing the midline—moving the eyes, hands, and arms over the midline of the body to the other side. Without this ability, even reading or writing is much more difficult, and children who are observed moving the whole body at a time often have difficulties with reading.

Rotation would be unthinkable without a sense of balance. Therefore, the foundation of our ability to balance is also part of the Lateral Family. For children who have problems with this, reading is not a favorite activity as it requires the eyes to go back and forth across the midline of sight. Eye–hand coordination is also important for catching a ball and is more difficult with a poor sense of balance.

Another aspect supported by the development of the Lateral Family is the ability to be with other people, to take someone under one's wing, and equally, when necessary, give them a prod with the elbow. Here in child development we see the Lateral Family as part of the foundation for unfolding willpower, characterized by defiant phases, discovering the word "no," and outbursts of rage in the supermarket with toddlers—until, by school age, it is hoped the capacity has developed to agree with others and compromise in one's own ideas.

PHASE 2: THE SIX *KEIRAKU*

After the Three Families have had a chance to develop and mature in a child, we can see the second phase emerge once the child is able to stand upright and walk freely. This is a transitional stage as the child goes from being mobile on all fours to two feet. The Three Families are now ready to transition to the next stage where they will differentiate further to support the upright position of a child. Here we see the directional qualities of traditional Japanese and Chinese medicine—the *yin* and *yang* meridians.

Yin and *yang* are a concept of Eastern traditions which we will not elaborate on in this book. For our purposes here, we can summarize that they are opposite qualities in the *Ki* (life force) that exist in harmony with one another and create balance in their flow against and in and out of one another. *Yin* energy in the human body travels upward from the earth toward the sky, and the *yang* energy in the body travels downward from the sky towards the earth. Each of the 12 primary meridians is *yin*-dominant or *yang*-dominant. The meridians form pairs in the Five Elements, which means that each one of the Five Elements has oppositional forces that flow upwards and downwards, giving the human body the ability to move in an upright position on the earth.

The ability for a child to stand upright and walk freely requires balance between the upward and downward energy in the meridians; this is Phase 2 of meridian development, when the Three Families further differentiate into the long meridians called the Six *Keiraku*.

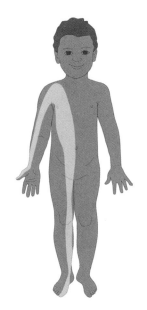

Spleen–Lung meridian

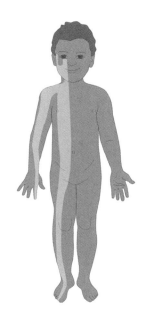

Stomach–Large Intestine meridian

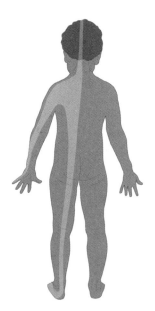

Bladder–Small Intestine meridian

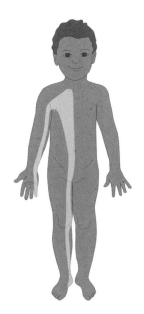

Heart–Kidney meridian

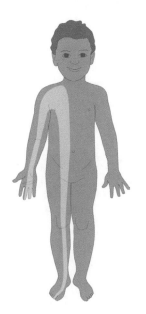 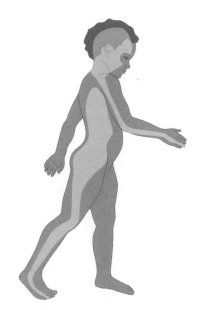

Liver–Pericardium meridian   *Gall Bladder–Triple Heater meridian*

This initial transition from the crawling position to standing on two feet does not mean the child is fully coordinated and balanced in the pelvis; he is still in the exploratory stage of the upright position and being able to walk without assistance. This whole new view from the child's eyes offers so much more stimulus that often a child doesn't know where to begin exploring! This is the basis for many round-about and defiant behaviors as the child turns back and forth away from the caregivers, often called rapprochement in developmental psychology.

This phase of the Six *Keiraku* brings a whole new orientation of the meridians. The meridians of one arm and one leg on the same side of the body are combined. In this way, up–down connections called the six axes in Japanese literature develop within the Three Families. The connections are between Stomach and Large Intestine meridians; Lung and Spleen meridians; Bladder and Small Intestine meridians; Kidney and Heart meridians; Gall Bladder and Triple Heater meridians; and Pericardium and Liver meridians.

At this stage of development, motor development is one of the main themes for preschool-age children as they are learning to master the body in every way they can. Anyone who is familiar with this stage of development in children knows the intense urge they have to move, explore, and be spontaneous in all of their emotions and desires in life. Conflicts are still acted out with hands-on resolution skills, and children have the urge to hit, slam, fondle, drop, and completely explore the spontaneous nature to move the energy expanding within them.

Children between the ages of two and three years who have learned to walk and run develop a new relationship with their environment. New needs and wants appear and seek fulfillment. Skills with the fingers and hands are improving, which is known to have a direct effect on a child's linguistic abilities. With increasing ability to manage and use the body, a child learns to make things happen in the world and so-called self-efficacy develops.

A child's movements during the *Keiraku* stage of development gradually become better coordinated. Walking, running, stopping suddenly, changing directions or speed if an obstacle gets in the way, balancing while climbing—all of these are gradually developing over the four- to six-year period. Games that involve running and catching, scooters, riding a bicycle, and playing on a swing are examples of motor skills that are being supported in the development of the *Keiraku* constellation. A child can coordinate movement not only in the activities mentioned above but also, for example, when walking at the same time as carrying a glass of water.

The *Keiraku* stage is also affected by interaction with the environment as children want to explore their impact on the world around them. They want to act upon, and satisfy, all of their curiosities. They are learning to regulate the body in relation to events going on around them, so as to be able to deal with them appropriately and efficiently. This means that children are learning to use only as much energy as necessary. They are also learning how to release tension through relaxation and, if necessary, hold energy in readiness for action.

Overall, a child is becoming better acquainted with her own body, with its reactions, needs, and sensations, and as she is doing this a foundation of her personal underlying condition of relaxation is developing. The way the environment allows a child to come back to a state of relaxation will affect a certain foundation of the whole wellbeing of the child later in life. Feelings, thoughts, experiences, environmental stimuli, other people, and all situations encountered have an effect on this underlying condition which can be seen in the developing muscle tone of a child, called tonus.

Many children come out of the Three Families phase with a state of tension that is already high. They have had experiences where their needs were either not met or were not taken seriously and respected. This can impair their capacity to show their feelings at this young age. Or the opposite may be the case: a state of resignation has set in, expressed in either slack or very tight muscle tone. Outwardly, this can show itself in awkward, faltering movements.

Learning to recognize one's own feelings and those of others is a distinguishing feature of the *Keiraku* stage. Children's feelings can differ widely in intensity, covering the full bandwidth from quiet sulking to rage. A child looks to her parents for confirmation that what she is feeling and expressing is OK, and this has a wide range of possibilities and growth between the ages of one and seven.

For example: a child has tripped and hurt herself. In the middle of the first sob, she seeks contact with her parents: "Am I—are my feelings—being taken seriously?" First, all she wants is confirmation—"Yes, that hurt!"—and then, second, she wants to be comforted. Yet how often is a child in today's world told "Oh, it didn't really hurt!" or "Don't make such a fuss!"?

If the child has this sort of experience over and over again in many situations in life, sooner or later the time comes when the child no longer risks expressing her feelings and those feelings can become more and more repressed.

The opposite is true when the underlying state of tension in the muscle tone of a child is flexible: there are more possibilities for a child to respond to her surroundings with many different patterns of movement—physically, cognitively, and emotionally.

When a child is given room to learn what feelings are and allowed to take them seriously, she can develop resiliency for challenges later in life. The *Keiraku* phase of development is the ground for this learning to happen.

Practice of feelings and emotions comes through squabbling, making friends, and experiencing frustrations. Here the child has to learn to get along with her own needs and those of others. Reconciliation following an argument, giving up something that one would like to keep, apologizing if one is in the wrong—these are the steps practiced and learned during the *Keiraku* stage. It is important for parents to allow their children to experience these challenges, giving them the chance to develop skills and strategies for action.

During this phase of development, motor development and all the themes linked with it are in the foreground. It is clear that the development of the meridians is very closely tied to movement. This also means that the less children move, the more the development of the meridians and their role in later life will be delayed. A child must reach a level of maturity in energetic development in order to go on to the next phase. This next level and phase corresponds to being ready to enter school, somewhere between six and seven years old.

Before starting school, however, other social skills need to develop. Social competence has to mature, and this means that there needs to be a more differentiated and controlled interaction between "I" and "you" (or the environment). As a more differentiated and controlled emotional expression evolves, a further pairing of meridians takes shape, along with readiness for school. This developmental stage is marked by the emergence of the Five Elements—the subject of this book.

PHASE 3: THE FIVE ELEMENTS

Once the up–down connection of the Six *Keiraku* has matured with the physical ability to move in the world in more coordinated and complex ways inwardly and outwardly from a sensorimotoric to a psychological way, an additional constellation of meridians has formed connecting the inner–outer reality for a child. The energetic system now has differentiated into the 12 primary meridians, linking the energy pathways to the skin, muscles, sinews, organs, tissues, brain, and cognitive/emotional processes. This is the point at which a child has reached the level of the Five Elements.

The development of the inner–outer connection in the meridian system now offers more awareness and fine-tuning abilities to work with emotional expressions. A child is now capable of developing individual reaction patterns and responses to different situations in life. This is different to the ability of the Six *Keiraku* to express emotions, where a child's capacity is limited more to direct, unfiltered expressions of emotions. When a child reaches the developmental stage of the Five Elements, the full *yin/yang* pairing of meridians has developed and offers more strategies for resolution and the development of more complex responses to emotions and conflicts in life. The capacity for abstract thinking develops more and more. The world is perceived in more multifaceted ways and comprehended in a way that is more differentiated.

A sign for a child reaching the developmental stage of the Five Elements will reflect an ability to express emotions in a manner that is adequate for a given situation. A child also has the ability to set aside his own needs during lessons in school and can pay attention for longer periods of time. A child that has entered into the Five Elements also demonstrates an ability to build friendships in the new environment of school, and to process the loss of old friends from kindergarten. When a child is able to do this, he is demonstrating the necessary social competencies to be ready for school. When a child has the ability to restrain himself, he usually has what is needed to learn how to write because even movement needs developmentally to be able to restrain itself or put the brakes on. A good example of this physical movement is writing the figure 8.

On the physical plane, a change of teeth also occurs during this phase. The number of teeth increases and the new teeth are bigger than the old ones. This allows for a firmer bite, which includes "setting one's jaw"—showing increased powers of assertiveness and perseverance.

The following is an overview of the energetic development phases:

- Energetic development happens in three big phases that merge fluidly one into another.

- Phase 1 corresponds to the developmental stage of the Three Families. This begins before birth and lasts until the child starts to walk.

- Phase 2 corresponds to the developmental stage of the Six *Keiraku*. This begins at the point where the child is standing up and walking, and at the end of kindergarten leads into the next phase.

- Phase 3 is the inner–outer linking of the 12 meridians—the Five Elements. This begins as the child reaches school age, somewhere between six and seven years old.

Each of these developmental phases lays the foundation for the next one and continues to exist as the foundation. This means that during any situation in life that we struggle to move through, we can refer back to the corresponding developmental themes. If one developmental stage has not unfolded adequately before transition into the next, we will always have a bit more difficulty with the subject area of the incompletely developed phase, even if it doesn't turn into a genuine stumbling block.

From the point of view of energetic development, many of today's school children are still at the kindergarten stage, or the end of the *Keiraku* stage of development. This means that emotional and social development are also lagging behind, as these are closely tied in with motor development. The children behave in a way that is fully appropriate for the developmental stage they are at, except that this developmental stage is not what is expected of a school child.

For this reason, in each of the Five Elements chapters in this book (Chapters 4–8), motor exercises are described to help with more precise observation and recognition of the developmental stage a child is at. The suggested games and activities can support children's further development. The purpose of working with the Five Elements is not to produce a perfect child or to eliminate particular behaviors in a child which others do not like. Rather, the purpose is to offer children an environment with more possibilities to express all of the Five Elements so that they can develop their innate strength and resiliency to grow and learn.

POSSIBLE PITFALLS OF THE ENERGETIC APPROACH

Using the three phases of energetic development to diagnose from a Western perspective, which categorizes children and pigeonholes their struggles into one phase or energetic level, is contrary to the whole Eastern view of energy. The holistic view of the energetic approach continually seeks to understand that who a child is and what they are experiencing in this moment is not a fixed expression of one of the phases. It is a pivotal opportunity to change what is struggling and seeking balance. This allows the grace of the innate nature of the energy in a child to reveal what it needs to move and grow.

For this reason, it is important to be very wary of any form of typification, or classifying a child into a diagnosable imbalance of one particular phase or stage. Typifying does create a kind of order, but it does so at the risk of clouding the image and respectful view of the individual child, especially when changes occur in the child and she is moving more freely once again in a particular stage or phase of energetic development.

When we typify, as a rule we formulate bias, deficits, and deviations from the norm, and not much range remains for individuality and particularities. The point of the Five Element view is to identify a child's opportunities and capabilities as the starting point. What matters is to observe the diverse characteristics, the uniqueness, and the multifaceted nature of each and every child.

Unfortunately, however, very often the practice of Eastern knowledge and the theory of the Five Elements is converted into a Western way of thinking. Examples of this are the many personality tests in popular magazines, where the answers to a few questions are supposed to reveal what "type" we are, and what we should do in this or that situation. The problem of typification is a recurring topic for discussion in professional development for therapists with Western training, and shows how difficult it is to transplant Eastern thought into our Western-trained heads.

When we observe children, we get a wealth of information. Here, the Five Elements are a great help in finding some order for it all, or finding an orientation. Out of the many mosaic fragments that we have gathered, there emerges an overall picture that enables us to get a sense of what gives a child's being its own particular stamp in each of the Five Elements. This requires great openness and freedom from bias on the part of the observer. It means, above all, not adopting a fixed view based on preliminary information, because every child continues to grow and develop expressions of the Five Elements when given the opportunity. It is important not to be tempted to try to fit a child into the Five Elements as though they are a rigid classification system.

When working with the energetic development phases with children, we challenge every hypothesis we use when describing children. This means we recognize that whatever we discern a child needs when working with them, the language itself tends to sound like we are using generalizations. We practice mindfulness and respect, remembering that the work itself is about the movement and constant change that we are supporting in a child's development.

When observing the energetic expressions of a child's development we are not looking for deficits and deviations from a norm, we are focusing on what a child is expressing now and what they have integrated and learned so far in the phases. It is important to recognize that a school-aged child's personality has been formed so far by the totality of their propensities in the Five Elements, their earlier development in the first two phases, and the environment that interacted and supported them in these stages of life. Additionally, every child is created at conception with their own unique energetic signature that will also affect how they respond to their environment and give them certain strengths or weaknesses in the Five Elements. This is why each child will develop their own individual characteristics and patterns of attitudes and reactions, which are visible in the motor, sensory, cognitive, and emotional expressions in life.

Mindfulness, respect, and attention to the development and personality of each and every child are the pillars of our work. Transposing the Five Elements into everyday life with children—be that in a therapy session, kindergarten, school, or at home—is an aid to their keeping, or recovering, their inner balance. In working and being with children, getting to know the Five Elements and their particular qualities is a valuable resource for approaching children's individual needs and abilities, so that we can create better environments for them to grow and develop into who they are destined to be in the world.

CHAPTER 2

The Foundation of
the Five Elements

As we begin the discussion that will deepen our understanding of the Chinese and Japanese Five Elements, we are faced with a small dilemma. Here, we are given the task of describing the identifiable stages of something that may appear to be five separate, isolated phases of the life force. But the truth about these energetic qualities is that they are a continuous, natural cycle that can only be understood if the movement and flow from Element to Element are acknowledged and applied.

We can understand this more easily if we use the language of analogy from which the Five Elements are derived. The Five Elements have a metaphorical relationship to the seasons of the planet, and they are called by the names Wood, Fire, Earth, Metal, and Water. They express the relationship of our existence with nature and have direct correspondences to the seasons: Spring, Summer, Indian Summer, Autumn, and Winter.

Time is a continuous loop. There is no real beginning or end as we move from year to year; only the changes of the seasons that create distinctions in time allow us to recognize that there is a repeating cycle. Each season will follow the next as long as our planet revolves around the sun. Likewise, each elemental phase will follow the next as long as life exists on the planet.

Each season is dependent on every other season. A farmer is dependent on nature to balance the environmental conditions of each season. If winter is too long, then springtime may be shortened, not giving enough time for planting crops or allowing new plants to mature before the sun's heat comes in the summer. If new buds are withered by too much heat, then crops will produce less food and there will be less seed to sow for the following year. Extra work may be required to prepare fields in the autumn for winter crops or springtime planting, and there will be less food available to store for surviving the winter months. Everything in nature affects the farmer's life, from the length of the seasons to the weather conditions each one brings. The seasons' continuous cycle affects every year in the future.

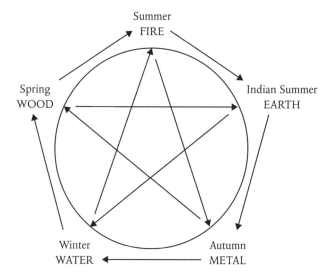

The cycle of the Five Elements and their correspondences with the seasons

In the same way, the Five Elements support the development of a human being. Every Element is affected by the one before and will affect the one that follows. Too much of one will take away from another, and the whole balance of development will be shifted.

The following is a brief description of the Five Elements and their analogous relationship to the seasons, nature, and developmental characteristics of humans.

The Five Elements

- The *Wood Element* represents the season of Spring. In the spring, life is bursting with growth and new life as seeds sprout from the ground and buds push out from the branches of trees and plants. Life stretches out and grows as fast and far as it can reach. In the human life cycle, Wood represents birth and growth—the times in life that are bursting with new energy, discovery, and movement. In every stage of our life, Wood is the energy that allows us to plan, create, and make decisions. It gives us flexibility, vision, and the emotion of anger when life doesn't manifest the way we envision it should. Wood expressions in the body relate to the ligaments, tendons, and sinews, giving us our flexibility on all levels in life.

- The *Fire Element* represents the season of Summer. In the summer, life is full of activity and vitality. The climate is hot and nature is at its peak of reproduction. Everything seems to communicate life in its full spectrum with whatever vigor is present. In the human life cycle, the Fire Element represents our young, reproductive, adult lives. Fire gives us the ability to be in relationships, and can be seen in our daily vitality, joy for living, and the energy for the expression of warmth and communication in our lives. Fire allows us to be open to all circumstances in life, joyous or sad, and rules the heart and circulatory system.

- The *Earth Element* represents the season of Indian Summer. It is the time of year in between summer and autumn, and also the short phase in between all seasons when the planet expresses more than one season at a time. Traditionally, this time of year is for harvesting, sowing seeds, collecting and distributing the bounty of the harvest, and storing it for the winter months ahead. It is the middle-aged stage of life, where we naturally "digest" and ponder on our life experiences, grounding our past into nutrition for the future. Earth is the energy in our daily activities that allows us to make life round and full. We can see the Earth Element characteristics in our digestion and whatever centers us, nurtures us and others, and allows us to stand in our opinions and truths while still maintaining compassion for others with different views in life. The Earth Element rules the tone of the flesh.

- The *Metal Element* represents the season of Autumn. Life on earth has the appearance of preparing for death in autumn. The winds begin to blow, the leaves change color and fall from the trees, the climate gets drier, and the moisture in nature withdraws inward toward the earth. The Metal Element represents old age in life, where the sage within us rules with deep reflections. This Element gives us the energy to take life's experiences and sort out the sacred pieces from the non-essentials. It is the time in life when we let go of the old to make room for the new. Grief is its emotion as we let go of what is no longer needed. Here we create our physical and internal boundaries. Wherever deep respect and acknowledgment are needed or exist, the Metal Element is present. Metal rules the skin, lungs, and the nose.

- The *Water Element* represents the season of Winter. Nature has the appearance of death in this season where the trees, shrubs, and earth appear barren. We know that winter is really a period of hibernation for the earth and many of her creatures. It is a time of rejuvenation, deep rest, and powerful stillness preparing for the bursting energy of new life again in spring. In the cycle of our life, it is the time of death and the stages of unknowns in between the present and our next reality, whatever our beliefs may be. In our everyday activities, the Water Element represents our fluidity, steadfastness, calmness, and ability to stay with the unknowns we are facing in life. Fear is the emotion that arises when faced with the darkness of unexplored paths and unrevealed outcomes, and courage is the strength of the Water Element that appears in its resolute commitment to flow and bring fluidity to our lives. The Water Element rules our deepest, supporting, physical structure— the bones and bone marrow.

The Five Elements mirror our personal development. They reveal unfolding processes through balanced and imbalanced expressions of physical health, mental states, and emotional wellbeing. It is easiest to see this when we go through stressful times in our lives.

Everyone reading this book can create a personal list of physical, mental, and behavioral responses they have when under stress. Some of us may eat too much, or we may have no appetite at all. Our skin may break out, become dry, or get rashes. Moods and behavior can vary from controlling and easily frustrated to withdrawn and on the verge of tears. Any of the characteristics listed in the Five Element descriptions above that we experience as dominating our behavior during times of stress, or which we are incapable of expressing, is pointing to potential imbalances in our personal development in the Five Elements.

In Chapter 1, we discussed how the energetic system unfolds through various stages of development as a child matures and how the movement of *Ki* is the precursor to sensory and motor development. An analogy often used to understand this is to look at the energy system as an amoeba-like field that is part of a developing child and human being. When a child is born, that amoeba is malleable and fluid, responding to the environment and itself, shape-shifting to whatever way is needed to survive and exist harmoniously in the world. As the amoeba-like field responds to repeated stimuli, healthy or unhealthy, it gets imprinted or fixated in its responses and a pattern of the same shape begins to form in other similar situations in life for survival. In this way, we see repeated patterns of behavior and physical symptoms to stressors in life, and these become more pronounced and predictable the longer one is exposed to stressors without being offered new stimuli or experiences to learn new patterns and responses. In this way, the energetic system can be seen as a buffer and support to a developing child and a continuous field that offers the possibility for change throughout a lifetime.

By the age of five to seven years, a child has the potential to have developed all 12 of the primary meridians in the Five Elements. These are the pathways that channel the *Ki* and assist the development of the expressions of the Five Elements. Each meridian is associated with one of the Five Elements, and they are represented in partnerships of *yin* and *yang* in each Element. This is how the physical functions of the body become connected to the Five Elements. The chart below shows some of the physical expressions of the body in relation to the meridians and their corresponding elemental phases.

The physical expressions of the Five Elements

The Five Elements	Wood	Fire	Earth	Metal	Water
Corresponding meridians	Gall Bladder and Liver meridians	Heart, Small Intestine, Triple Heater, and Pericardium meridians	Spleen and Stomach meridians	Lung and Large Intestine meridians	Bladder and Kidney meridians
Sensory organ	Eyes	Tongue	Mouth and pharynx	Nose	Ears
Sensory function	Vision, seeing	Speech	Taste	Smell	Hearing
Bodily fluids	Tears	Blood and sweat	Saliva for digestion	Mucus	Saliva or lubrication
Tissue and body parts	Ligaments and tendons	Blood vessels	Connective tissue, fatty tissue	Skin, mucous membranes	Bones, teeth, and bone marrow
Tastes	Sour desires/ dislikes	Bitter desires/ dislikes	Sweet desires/ dislikes	Spicy and pungent desires and dislikes	Salty desires and dislikes
External, physical expression of the Elements	Nails	Complexion and face color	Lips	Skin and body hair	Hair on the head, teeth
Smells from the body	Rancid	Burnt	Sickly sweet	Rotten	Putrid
Verbal expression of the Elements	Yelling, shouting	Lively, expressive, laughing	Singing tone of voice	Nasal, whining	Sighing, moaning

What information can we draw from the chart? What do these correspondences actually mean?

The energetic system is an amazing choreography of the dance between the physical and non-physical concepts we are using in our Five Element work with children. The chart above gives us information about these two realities and clues to other levels of development that we will be observing later in children. A child who craves sweets or avoids them all of the time is pointing to a possible imbalance in the Earth Element at that moment. Or a child with chronic congestion or intestinal viruses is showing signs of potential imbalances in the Metal Element at that moment. These correspondences are like a roadmap to children's development and offer us tools to observe, work, and play with their unfolding processes of growth and learning.

The Five Elements in Child Development

The descriptions below are a generalized overview of some of the specific developmental characteristics that each elemental phase is responsible for in the natural development of a child when they reach the maturity of stepping into the Five Element developmental stage. This condensed explanation reveals the energetic role of the Five Elements at play in the physical, emotional, social, and psychological development of all human beings.

- The *Wood Element* provides the foundation for the development of all movement. The ability to move in this world is a learning process that requires coordination and planning. We can observe Wood Element expressions in children through their ability to plan and coordinate their own movements. These early planning strategies develop into the ability to focus on the movement of objects and later the ability to direct imaginary games with friends. The development of large motor skills is an expression of the Wood Element.

- The *Fire Element* is expressed in the experience of togetherness and the feeling of "us." Fire is seen in the development of partnerships and the ability to form relationships. The first developing relationships we observe in an infant is with the parents. Fire can also be seen in a child's vitality, joy, and enthusiasm for life. The development of speech and all levels of communication are expressions of the Fire Element.

- The *Earth Element* is distinguishable when a child expresses a strong ability to concentrate. A child who appears to be at home in herself regardless of her surroundings, and develops an ability to be alone at age-appropriate lengths, is displaying Earth Element characteristics. A centeredness, sense of gravity, balance, and the ability to stand strong in one's own views are strong expressions of the Earth Element. Digestion, appetite, and the way a child receives nourishment early in life and creates nourishment for the self later in life are also developments from the Earth Element.

- The *Metal Element* expresses itself in the development of self-perceptions and boundaries. Early characteristics are visible in the capacity of a child to be touched or held. Our first development of self-awareness is through the skin. Later developments appear in a child's social competence as the ability to express respect for others' boundaries and to create self-boundaries. The Metal Element develops the capacity for acceptance, tolerance, respect, and appreciation.

- The *Water Element* is expressed in a readiness and ability to move into new situations in life. Early characteristics can be seen in a child's ability to rest deeply regardless of changes in his environment. An overall calm demeanor when undertaking any task accompanied by patience and steadfastness is the advanced expression of this quality. The courage to enter something new finds its expression here. This capacity to move into new situations in life takes an ability to listen, relax, and be silent enough to come into contact with one's own depth. Good fine motor skills are also a strong Water Element capacity.

These characteristics reveal to us the ways the Five Elements can unfold their development in balanced expressions. If a child is able to develop in all of the levels described above, he will have a great head start in life. Such a child would likely become a very talented adult with the ability to express himself professionally and personally in many ways. The more expressions the Five Elements learn, the more the energy of each Element is available to keep expanding and offering new possibilities of responses to situations in life.

Anyone who has had the opportunity to observe children grow through various stages of their life would probably agree that it is a rare occurrence to witness a development like this. It is natural for children to experience difficulties in different stages of their life, and it is part of the task of the Five Elements to help children discover new ways to move through unbalanced stages of their development.

Imagine the following five examples of children in a kindergarten class:

---

1. Five-year-old Kathy does not like to move around very much in her kindergarten classroom. When she has to take part in activities that require large motor skills, she is very anxious and over-cautious. Her movements are slow and contemplated 10–15 times before she participates in physical skills and activities. Most of the time, she plays in a self-absorbed way in the doll corner of the classroom, and when other children take her toys, she does not try to defend what she is playing with.

2. Eight-year-old Sebastian has a recognizable stuttering pattern that began when he was three. He used to be a very vivacious child with a lot of friends, but now in school he withdraws into himself more and more to get away from the danger of being talked to. His joy and playfulness have diminished and he appears sad most of the time.

3. It is impossible for Nicholas to wait his turn when the class is doing activities. By the time the second or third person has a turn, he forgets completely his place in line and rushes forward to take a turn. Once he has started the project, he loses interest within 5–10 minutes. It is difficult for him to finish any project without the assistance of a teacher. He is

also easily influenced by others' creativity and quickly leaves his own ideas to follow someone else's plan.

4. Little Josh is not interested in any tactile activities such as playing in the sandbox and baking sand cookies in his kindergarten class. He avoids hugging and cuddling from his mother and she often feels rejected.

5. Five-year-old Catherine always feels as if she has to use the toilet without any real need. Her teachers comment that when she is doing a project, she is incredibly persistent, patient, and steady, no matter how long it takes or how many times she has to repeat the steps to complete the activity.

All of these children are experiencing difficulties in expressing one or more of the Five Elements. The Wood Element is Kathy's most difficult phase; this shows in her lack of development in motor skills, coordination, and decision making. Sebastian shows Fire Element imbalances with his stuttering, lack of joyfulness, and avoidance of playing with other children. Nicholas's Earth Element is struggling as he demonstrates difficulties in staying focused, completing activities, and staying with his own ideas in crafts. Josh avoids stimulation to the skin and contact that would allow him to feel his own boundaries; therefore the Metal phase calls our attention. Catherine shows the steadfast characteristics of Water, but the constant sensation to urinate without real need shows that there is an inner tension and persistence that does not allow true relaxation in the flow and process of what she is doing. Here we come back to the two basic questions we asked in the introduction to this book:

1. "Is this the way these children are choosing to act, or is this the only behavior they are capable of at this time?"

2. "*What* is this child expressing at this time, and why isn't he or she capable of more?"

From the Five Element perspective, these children are not *choosing* to act this way. These are their natural responses to the total environment in their lives. They are expressing the Elements' struggle to move and develop. How they will be able to continue developing more advanced expressions of these Elements as they grow will depend on how their environment responds and supports the difficult stages that they are now in.

When children are born into this world, they are born with their senses wide open. They are unable to protect themselves from the highly advanced technology and fast-paced lifestyles that consume our families today. Invasive and unnatural influences that do not offer healthy Five Element environments can disturb the fragile inner balance of a newborn and begin to alter the flow of energetic development. This can happen again and again as a child continues to grow. From school settings, to local media, to new or older siblings, or to simple misunderstandings of a child's intention to express himself, repeated responses from the world that do not understand a child's developmental needs can create limitations in the natural flow and development of the Five Elements. A child will express himself with what he has learned or how he has been allowed to develop, and will not take on new forms of behavior or responses unless given the right stimulus to move in a new way.

Thus, we observe energetic development as the precursor to all other levels of development. Our experience shows us that perception and development challenges stem from an energetic basis. Therefore, a balance in the Five Elements is a needed support for the development of all other capabilities.

Our search for a way to find the right forms of stimulus to open and balance the flow of the Five Elements in children is where the Five Element work began and what the "Room to Play" children's therapy in Germany was based on. The work looked closely at our second question: "*What* is this child expressing at this time, and why isn't he or she capable of more?" Here, attention was called to children like Nicholas, the kindergarten boy who couldn't remember that he had to wait his turn and would constantly rush to the front of the line. The consequence was that he ended up consistently at the end of the line. Why did this boy continually "forget" and repeat a behavior that was counter-productive to what he wanted?

After watching many children like Nicholas, with numerous varieties of struggling expressions of the Five Elements, it became clear to us that the Elements have a drive to grow. It is the nature of the life force to express itself. Children who repeat counter-productive behavior patterns are crying out for help to move what is innate within them by continually expressing the level to which they have developed.

The next chapters will explore more deeply the expressions of the Five Elements in life, and the ways in which the Five Element work is a process of offering opportunities for balancing this natural cycle. What we have discovered in this healing process is that the more a child has the opportunity to express and develop all of the Five Elements, the greater her chance for a round and full development. An inner harmony arises when each of these elemental phases finds room to grow, and in turn allows children to grow closer to themselves, to people, and to the world they live in.

PART II

The Five Elements in Child Development

CHAPTER 3

The Five Elements
Wood, Fire, Earth, Metal, and Water

The Five Elements develop slowly over time within each one of us. Their cycles and presence are innate and unfold a very personal expression of who we become in this world. Western medicine explains through genetics that our physical characteristics and propensities are given to us by our parents. As described in Chapter 1, Eastern medicine has a similar belief, with the added concept of a life force that the Japanese call *Ki*. The *Ki* is an individual energy we are born with that fuels all of our development and life-sustaining abilities until the day we die. At the moment of conception, our individual *Ki* begins its path of unfolding. Our constitutional propensities for physical, mental, psychological, and spiritual expressions are determined by the state of our parents' *Ki*.

It is important to understand that when we speak of the "constitutional propensities" of *Ki*, it does not mean that our personality and health are predetermined. On the contrary, these propensities merely give us tendencies toward certain expressions of the *Ki* as it develops in response to the environment around us. Our adult expression of physical and mental health is created from our ability to respond to what we encounter growing up. The patterns in adult physical, mental, and emotional expressions are the outcome of how the individual *Ki* adapted to the environments it was exposed to since conception.

As discussed in the section on energetic development in Chapter 1, the initial development of the *Ki* in a fetus is dependent on the mother's health and the environment she lives in. Many of us have heard relatives speak about family resemblances in the way a newborn or baby reacts to sound, temperature, or movements in their surroundings. They may be describing early visible propensities of the constitution of the *Ki*. As a child continues to grow and is exposed to more and more experiences in the physical, mental, and emotional environments—air, climate, food, water, textures, space to move, the emotional and psychological interactions of others— her overall energetic development will continue to be affected. The *Ki* is malleable in nature and will continue to respond to the total surroundings of a child, laying the foundation for her personal expressions of the Five Elements later in life.

A very simple example of this in our modern world could occur when a child conceived by parents living in Alaska relocates to Florida. Depending on how many generations this child's family has lived in a cold climate, and how old the child is when arriving in Florida, her life energy will respond and develop differently than if she were raised in Alaska.

The differences in the seasons between Alaska and Florida would be a shock to anyone's system. However, in a child, the *Ki* has not yet developed a variety of ways to adapt to extreme changes in environment. The effects of the shock on the life force may show up in more pronounced ways in a child than it would in an adult because adults have experienced more situations in life that required them to cope with changes and have developed the capacity to respond with various expressions in all of the Five Elements. A child under five or six years of age has not yet developed distinctions in all of the Five Elements. Signs of a child's *Ki* struggling to adapt to this example of a very different environment could appear in sleep pattern difficulties, an inability to relax or feel at ease, or reluctance in making new friends and going into new play settings without a parent's presence. It is very common for children who are experiencing difficulties like these to be in a developmental stage where the *Ki* is limited in its response to an environment and struggling to find new ways to adapt. This can sometimes appear as regressed behaviors in children as they step backwards to what the *Ki* does know in how to respond to the different environments.

The way in which the parents and significant adults respond to the behavioral, physical, and developmental difficulties a child expresses will deeply affect the child's ability to adjust and grow in the new environment. This example is a drastic demonstration of how changes in the environment can affect the expressions of the *Ki*, which is the foundation of the development of the Five Elements in our lives. It is helpful to know that all children go through many changes and transitions, and need to go through these changes to develop. New siblings, new homes, new friends, new caretakers, and new schools all offer developmental opportunities for a child's constitutional propensity to interact with the environment and find new ways to respond so that the overall growth can develop into a broad range of expressions in the Five Elements.

What we are describing is not new or beyond most people's insights into the developmental challenges children go through. Most reading this book will find much of this to be common sense. What we are offering is a possibility to observe the natural phenomena of development through an ancient and archetypal pattern that not only validates what you already know but also offers more ideas for how to respond directly to difficulties children encounter as they grow. By understanding the expressions and patterns of the Five Elements, we can see more clearly what children are asking for in their development when they are struggling and support them with more appropriate experiences to grow and develop.

This is one of the gifts of the unfolding development of the *Ki*. Children have the opportunity to develop many expressions of the Five Elements if given the right stimulation and room to play with their responses to life. The innate nature of the Five Elements is to find movement and growth, regardless of an individual's propensities, and to continue this expansion throughout the course of a lifetime. The Five Elements are developed at an elementary level and are available for children somewhere between the ages of five and seven years old.

Elementary expressions of the Five Elements must be given permission to occur in childhood in order for a child to develop balanced adult manifestations of the Five Elements. Knowing this helps us to understand the normalcy of temper tantrums, aggressive behaviors, fearful expressions, or any other behavioral "concerns" we often have about children acting out in various situations in life. We can begin to see that these behaviors in children are outlets to move something primal inside. This understanding gives us room to allow children to be children and to play with the many expressions that arise, as we look for how to offer new possibilities for the Elements to learn more ways to express themselves and grow.

The rest of this part is dedicated to describing each one of the Five Elements from the fully developed adult level of expression to the early and pre-elemental stages of expression in a developing child. The adult section will offer a guided imagery example of each Element; a description of the way each Element expresses itself fully in adult lives; and a chart with physical, seasonal, emotional, and cognitive correspondences of each Element in adult lives.

The children's section of each Element is more detailed in its description of what the early expressions of the Elements look like in balanced and imbalanced physical, behavioral, emotional, and psychological forms. Real-life examples of balanced and imbalanced children we have worked with over the years offer a view of the various ways we can see the Elements expressing themselves. Emphasis is also given to assessing whether a child has developed the foundation of the energetic road map to the early Five Element expressions. As described in Chapter 1, two other energetic stages must occur first—the Three Families and Six *Keiraku*. These two earlier stages must be stimulated and developed for a child to begin the elementary expression of the Five Elements and later advance into more mature adult expressions.

The end of each children's section offers an overview chart of the early balanced and imbalanced Five Element expressions in children; questions to help observe how your children are expressing each of the Elements at this time in their development; and a list of what the Element needs to mature and develop.

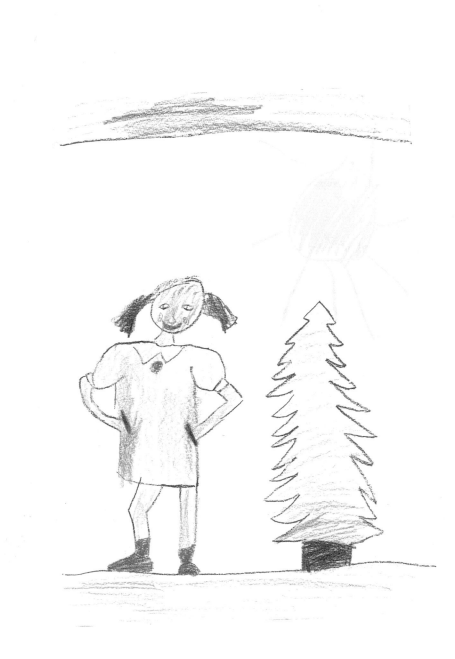

CHAPTER 4

The Wood Element in Child Development

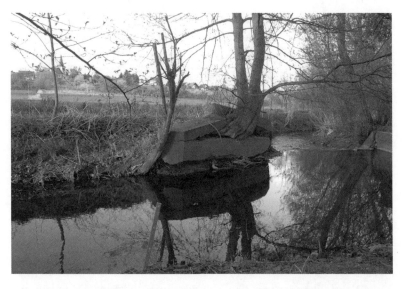

We would like to invite you to take part in a small experiment to get in the mood for the Wood Element. Wood signifies the need for discovery, growth, creativity, movement, and the desire for adventure. Make yourself comfortable and open your imagination as you read the following.

Adults

A Wood Element Experience

The winter has been long and hard, with bitter cold days that kept you huddled in your jacket when walking outside. Weeks of cloudy skies leave you feeling reluctant to open your eyes and greet the morning. But something feels different as you begin to rustle and stretch under the many layers of comforters in your warm bed. A small stream of light flickers from a crack in the blinds and your body feels a slight jolt as it recognizes the possibility of sunshine! Throwing back the covers, you jump out of bed to open the blinds and unveil the tease of the sunbeam. There in front of your eyes are the first signs of spring. Without thought, your body leaps with excitement and your limbs feel as though they are bursting with energy! Your body stretches with a "Yes!" and your mind shouts an "Aha!" as you glance at a flower poking out of the melting snow in front of your window. Tiny green sprigs reveal themselves on the shrubs and branches of the elm tree, and the street seems to have an excitement you haven't felt all winter.

Your mind races to the days ahead. Warm, sunny walks, jogging in the early morning, concerts, the smell of new grass, and even that project at work seem to have a new view. Full of ideas and a renewed sense, you prepare yourself for the day while writing down the plans that come popping into your mind. Life feels full of possibilities and you are eager to greet and start the day.

Expression of the Wood Element

The Wood Element gives us the energy to get out of bed in the morning with eagerness and gusto. With a strong, upright posture, flexible both internally and externally, we immerse ourselves in the day's tasks.

Wood gives us the capacity to develop the *artist, strategist,* and *planner* within. The *artist* gives us the new ideas and insights of what is needed to create the next moment in life. The *strategist* empowers us with a broad picture of the larger goals in our life, while the *planner* creates the details necessary to reach those goals. We can motivate others to work with us toward these larger goals. The *strategist* in us utilizes the right leadership qualities to inspire a team with our ideas and an ability to get others to collaborate wholeheartedly in realizing our goals. The *strategist* also gives us the capacity to keep the overall plan of the vision in view so that we can direct and coordinate the actions without losing control of the steps and details. The *artist* helps us to stay flexible when new ideas arise to keep the plan moving. We are clear and specific in our dealings with co-workers, but also considerate and open to other ideas.

It is easy for us to analyze the course of a project when the Wood Element is clear in us. We can keep a perspective of the original idea that gave birth to the project, how that project is capable of unfolding in the moment, and where we wish to go with it next to meet the desired outcome. The roles of creative director, planner, and overseer of projects are innate capacities for us in the Wood Element expression. When there is a conflict, it also allows us to manage anger or frustrations that may arise. It offers us the ability to have a clear picture of the essentials, recognizing problems so that we can utilize problem-solving skills. Through our capacity to plan broadly, we are in a position to measure our personal responsibilities, how much room we have to make decisions, and the time and money needed to complete the vision. The Wood Element gives us confidence in our personal originality; it continually redefines our claim to it, and it does not allow anyone to dispute our position.

On the following page is a chart of Wood Element expressions and some of their environmental, physical, behavioral, and psychological correspondences. Physical problems related to the areas of the body that the Wood Element governs in children or adults could be revealing the body's struggle with current life issues, constitutional propensities of the *Ki* when under stress, or constitutional limitations in handling different seasons or environmental conditions.

The behavioral and psychological expressions shown in the table correspond with Wood Element characteristics that are available for adults and some adolescents. Typically, pre-teens and teenagers are unpredictable and unstable in the consistency of these mature ranges of expressions in the Elements because their brain chemistry is in the process of changing during hormonal development. Adults interacting with teenagers should keep this in mind and be aware that it is normal for there to be large ranges of maturity in the expressions of the Elements from one teenager to the next, as well as within each teenager. Also, an encouraging note for us as adults when observing the Five Element expressions in ourselves and other adults is that they all still exist within us and hold the potential to move and develop more distinct and clear expressions in our lives.

Correspondences and characteristics of the Wood Element

Season	Spring
Climate	Windy
Tissue/body parts	Muscles, sinews, ligaments
Bodily fluids	Tears
Orifices	Eyes
Sensory organs	Eyes
Sensory function	Vision, seeing
Taste	Sour
External, physical form of expression	Nails
Balanced behavioral expressions	Assertive and confident; seeks challenges and adventure; readiness to take risks; loves movement and action; creative; good decision-making capacity with foresight and clarity; self-expressive
Behavioral expression under stress	Irritable, impatient, confrontational, arrogant, aggressive, over-controlling, emotional outbursts, wrathful, lack of vision in life or desire for growth, ambivalent, indecisive, compulsive, inability to make decisions, unclarity, timidity
Balanced physical expressions	Flexible, active
Imbalanced physical symptoms	Migraines, muscle spasms, vascular headaches; all eye problems; cracked, brittle, flaky nails; problems with joints, prone to tendon or ligament injuries; vertigo; lack of flexibility in muscles, stiffness, weak joints
Verbal expression	Clear, distinct, shouting
Strength	Capacity for control, self-control

Children
Expressions of the Wood Element

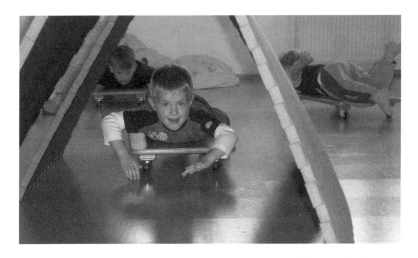

Much of childhood is Wood time. This is expressed through the love of movement, spontaneity, creativity, desire for adventure, and drive for discovery. Wood Element energy supports the process of growth and development. A child whose Wood aspect develops harmoniously is full of zest for action, sprouts new ideas, and is original. Within a group of children, she comes up with ideas and suggestions for games. She keeps a grasp of what's happening in the game and, like a little general, eagerly takes on leadership of the group. She has the big picture in front of her, a broader vision than others, and determines how everyone will march in a line. When Wood energy is balanced, the child can change roles and will join in another child's expanding vision with great enthusiasm, when she sees it's a better or more interesting one than her own. Yet, even in that circumstance of following others, clear Wood energy gives the child the ability to maintain her own creative input so that she does not disappear from the unfolding process of the game.

As the Wood Element develops in children, they learn to express what they need in their lives to grow and be creative. They have a directing energy that not only creates what is needed in the life space but also has the ability to resist confrontation and to defend or protect their "own realm."

Jocelyn was a creative, strong-minded little girl. She went through a phase at five-and-a-half years old when she would get up every morning and go immediately to the play room and sit down to draw—without a "hello," morning hug, or request for anything. Here, she would draw, paint, or color a picture for herself, and when finished would say, "Look what I did, Mommy!" Only after this was finished would she come into the kitchen for breakfast and continue on with the morning salutations and beginning of the day. When the mother tried to talk to Jocelyn before she drew in the morning, Jocelyn would ignore her, lightly push her away, or barely recognize she was being talked to. If the morning required a quick departure, Jocelyn would get angry and physically refuse to let her mother dress her. Eventually, the mother learned that she could have a happy start to days like this with her daughter if she brought a box of crayons and a notebook for the car on mornings that interrupted the five-year-old's ritual and need for creative expression first thing in the morning. When given this option, Jocelyn would cooperate and get ready to leave with her mother before her drawing time.

This is only one example out of a million possibilities of a young child directing what they need in their life to grow. Many see individual desires in children as obstinate or stubborn behaviors that cause alarm. How we react to these challenges in children can have a big effect on many levels as the Elements continue their physical, behavioral, emotional, and psychological development.

Imbalanced Expressions of the Wood Element

Difficulties in the Wood development of a 5–7-year-old, as well as adolescents and adults, could look like the child who sits "alone on a hill" and directs the group play "from the top down," wanting to take control without participating herself in the activity. Such a child will be furious when her plans are crossed by someone else. Children struggling in the development of Wood can appear to only know "Yes" or "No" ("If you're not for me, you're against me") as they lack the awareness of the notes in between, the shadings that can be useful in reaching a solution or a compromise with other children. The capacity of a child to reach a decision among many possibilities may be underdeveloped and show up with the need to over-control.

When plans do not go as wished in a child with unbalanced Wood energy, he may react with destructive behavior. A child like this could be aggressive and irritable, or could choose to no longer participate in the game at all. The "circus director," who must now relinquish his job to another child, is offended and cannot condescend under any circumstances to play the role of "clown" for even a moment. He would rather not play, or, full of anger, he may turn on another child and break his toys.

When Wood Element aspects of the *Ki* in a child are underdeveloped or suppressed, a child may be observed showing signs of indifference, lack of interest, or passivity. Moreover, this child may direct aggression against herself, which can, for example, be expressed bodily in nail-biting or pinching her own body. When told "No," the reaction is to be offended or sulky, or to make a dramatic scene. She assumes that all expressions of feeling and all reactions of others are about her, even when this is not the case. Yet, when her own living or play area is taken over by another child, she doesn't have the drive to protect it. On the contrary, she wouldn't harm even a fly. This holding back can lead to strains and cramps in the child, particularly in the head, neck, and shoulder regions. Cramped hands might be the proverbial clenched fists in the pocket. This cramping is an expression of powerlessness and displays itself also in restricted mobility. The gait of a child might be uncertain. The flow of movement could be hampered, faltering, or slowed down, and can appear angular and stumbling. A child like this might lack adeptness in gross motor activity and is deficient in movement skills. She may also have a restricted movement pattern that exhibits a lack of variation.

Although a child with unbalanced Wood struggles to gain dexterity of movement and tries repeatedly with perseverance, he does not succeed in carrying out the movement or does so only inadequately. Frequently, a child like this fails even at planning movement. Moreover, his ability to survey his surroundings with his eyes can often be limited because of weak or defective vision. Likewise, deficient spatial orientation and self-perception (self-image), as well as imprecise ideas about his own body and structure (body pattern), represent learning delays. The results are discouragement and deeper withdrawal from the surroundings, often with Wood Element imbalances.

Six-year-old Katrin (see below) is typical of children with disturbances in the Wood Element. It is not common to see as many capacities of an Element disturbed as is the case with Katrin. When this many facets of an Element are disturbed, it is the flag that points to the possibility that the first two developmental stages of the Three Families and Six *Keiraku* are not completed. When a large enough number of certain imbalanced characteristics appears in patterns like hers, it leads to judgments from society and children become labeled with names and categories. A child like Katrin is often called "ugly duckling" and "awkward," or even described as having two left feet. However, when the disharmony in the corresponding Element is recognized early on as a search and cry for balance, such children can be spared much suffering.

Katrin is very anxious and cautious in her movements and seeks to control precisely everything that she does. When running-type games or group games take place in kindergarten, she struggles to participate, because she cannot carry out all of the movements. Whatever group she plays in usually loses because of her, so she is unpopular as a group member, which makes her even more uncertain in herself and her movements. Although she would like to play along, she no longer joins in the games at the start, to avoid being disappointed.

In the doll corner, the teachers observe that when Katrin is playing with a toy, she readily lets another child take it away from her, even though she wants to play with it. To the other children, it's obvious that they can do whatever they want with Katrin.

Clearly, then, she appears to be excessively conforming, as she wants to avoid conflict. Even her slightest attempts to resolve a conflict are awkward and without a sense of self-worth. Occasional outbursts of aggressiveness are expressed in nail-biting.

Katrin is a typical example of a child who has not yet matured enough to be able to fully step into the Five Elements because she is still in the *Keiraku* phase of development. Katrin needs to focus so much energy on her motor skills that she doesn't have enough *Ki* to develop the qualities of the Wood Element.

Environmental Influences on the Development of the Wood Element

Infants come into contact with their surroundings and express themselves through movements. From nuzzling to suckling and following the eyes and faces of the parents and siblings, these early forms of movement are the foundation influencing the initial stages of all interaction and contact with the world. As a child grows, his self-concept is discovered and created through movement and interactions with his surroundings. Those surroundings are the initial environment and exposure to the Five Elements in the world and the direct way adults affect and support the overall development of a child.

In Wood, it is the caretaker's role to make sure the environment is safe and peaceful for the infant to grow and continue the natural need for movement and curiosity to discover. The way anger, conflict resolution, and shared planning are expressed in the environment of a child affects her development and the ways she is encouraged to engage in new activities and movements.

Learning agility of movement in new environments for a child creates a foundation for positive self-image on many levels. Gross motor skills with supple and flexible movements are supported when a child has permission from the environment to move and explore.

The ability to see and have visual awareness, to know that there is space around you, and the capacity to perceive your orientation in a room or to other objects are also dependent on the early development of movement. Overall, balanced Wood Element activities support the development of economical use of strength, good control of movement, and adaptive movement patterns that together produce coordinated, harmonious, physical behavior in a child.

When a child truly reaches the developmental capacity to begin developing the early expressions of the Wood Element, the *Ki* of

Wood gives the child an assertive ability to create and learn how to be flexible with others in the creative process. Wood offers the energy for learning how to lead and follow, to plan and carry out detailed tasks with others, and to develop problem-solving skills in conflicts.

The following exercises are ways to assess if a child is developmentally ready to focus fully on Wood Element development. In the above example, Katrin, a child with Wood imbalances, experienced a lot of difficulty with the exercises.

Talking with the mother, we found that the mother herself was anxious about movement. If Katrin wanted to climb or jump, the mother always stopped her because she was afraid that Katrin would hurt herself.

Getting both of them into more playful movement, and changing Katrin's room at home so that she was able to jump on an old mattress or swing on a special hanging mat, the *Keiraku* stage strengthened and the Wood Element was allowed to start growing. On this foundation it was then possible to start working more with the Wood Element.

Exercises
IS THE CHILD READY FOR WOOD ELEMENT DEVELOPMENT?

The behavior of Katrin is a perfect example of a good reason to assess whether a child is ready to begin working with exercises to develop the elementary expressions of the Five Elements or if they need to be assessed for their development of the *Keiraku*. As stated in the previous part of the book, the Three Families and the Six *Keiraku* lay the foundation for the unfolding of the Five Elements in a child's development. If these two stages of development are not complete, the unfolding of the elementary expressions of the Five Elements will be affected. When the Six *Keiraku* are not developed, a child will focus her energy on the development of motor skills for physical activities and have a limited amount of energy to develop the social, emotional, and cognitive abilities of the Five Elements.

This section offers movement exercises and questions to assess the development of the *Keiraku* in a child, followed by exercises for a child to help stimulate any underdeveloped *Keiraku* that becomes apparent. When there is a readiness for a child between the ages of five and six to begin developing the Wood Element expressions, he is able to perform these exercises. If a child has difficulty doing these exercises, it is possible to help the development of the Wood Element by integrating these exercises and games as much as possible in their daily lives.

Movement Exercises
1. Jumping Jack
The practitioner asks the child: "Do you know how to do a Jumping Jack? Try it, will you?" If the child hasn't got any idea of what to do, the practitioner should show the movements by doing them herself. Jump in the air with the legs wide apart, and at the same time clap your hands above your head. Then swing the arms down to the sides with the hands clapping on the thighs, as you bring your legs back together again.

QUESTIONS FOR ASSESSMENT

1. Can the child carry out the movements at least three times in succession?

2. Can he move his arms and legs in different ways at the same time?

3. Does he do the movements one after the other?

2. Lateral Jump
Place a rope about 16 inches in length on the floor, or draw a line on the floor the same length.

The practitioner says to the child: "Stand sideways (parallel) to the rope. Now, keeping your legs close together, jump over the rope as many times as you can in 15 seconds—keep jumping back and forth over the rope."

Before you start counting the jumps, five practice jumps are allowed. Jumps only count if they are done with the legs together and without touching the rope.

QUESTIONS FOR ASSESSMENT

1. Can the child do 15 jumps?

2. Do her feet stay together when she jumps?

3. Do her feet touch the line?

4. Does the child have to use her arms for support?

If you answered no to any of the questions in Movement Exercises 1 and 2, the following exercises can be done to help further the development of the *Keiraku* in a 5–7-year-old child.

Keiraku Development Exercises
1. As Strong as a Tree: Visualization for Children

a. "Imagine you are a tree. You've got firm roots reaching into the earth, and you're standing straight. You spread out your arms like branches. Now a light breeze is blowing and the tree starts moving in the wind, back and forth. The wind is also blowing from the side—how is the tree moving now? The wind is sometimes blowing from the front, and then from behind, and from one side, and then the other side—just try which kinds of movements the wind makes the tree move without falling over. Now get a piece of paper and draw your tree—what does it look like? What season is it and what kind of leaves does it have?"

b. Here is another idea: "Now you need a partner. Perhaps you'd like to ask a friend, your brother or sister, or your mother. One of you becomes the tree again. You have already tried out what the wind feels like. Now your partner is going to be the wind. He/she presses lightly once, in the front, on your breastbone (that's here [points]) and once from behind on your back. Do a quick and short press, and not too hard. See how it feels to resist against the press. Don't forget to take turns."

2. Now We Are Going to Japan (Idea for a Group)

a. "You already know that Japan is far away from here. How do you get there?" Get ideas from the children. Depending on their age, you might get a lot of funny ideas, such as walking, swimming, or going by car. Keeping the inquiry lighthearted and fun is part of relaxing into the movements needed for the *Keiraku*.

 Collect the children's ideas. Discuss together how to transfer the possible ways of traveling into movements. Ask what it is like to sit for a long time without moving if they haven't already made comments about that. Think of ways you can move on the airplane while you are traveling.

b. "Before boarding the airplane, all the joints in the body need to be moved. Stand up and move all the joints in your body." Allow the children's sense of silliness to come out as they wiggle and move all their joints in creative ways.

 "Now that we have moved all of our joints, press your right hand on your left knee and stretch your left arm towards the ceiling. Now, change to the other side, and now it's getting faster!"

 Repeat several times.

 "And now, while still standing, stretch both arms up to the ceiling, making yourself taller and taller, and then make yourself really small. And now, take a huge step with one foot to the right, and move both arms in a huge arc or half-circle above your head and to the same side; then to the left side. Do this back and forth."

 Repeat this several times.

 "Now, in the airplane, there is so little space that you can only move your feet. Still from a standing position, lift your heels off the floor and go up on to your toes very fast, three times! Great! You've reached your destination at last—get off the plane. To say 'hello' now, we bow to each other."

3. The World is Full of Colors

Each child sits down on a blanket and imagines that it's a big bath full of paint.

All the children can say which color they have chosen. Then, with each child twisting and rolling on their blanket, they can "paint" themselves in the color of their choice.

"Is every part of your body covered with paint? Good, now we're going to paint the floor!"

The children roll across the room. If they touch another child, the colors mix. Now what color can it be?

"So, now you're going to paint the soles of your feet—then, with big or little steps, you can make tracks all over the room!"

Finally, of course, all the children have to take a "shower." They find a place in the room and shake off the paint under the shower.

Overview

Expressions of the Wood Element in children

	Balanced expressions	Imbalanced expressions
Behavioral expressions	*The little leader* Goal-oriented, strategic thinker, seeks action, adventure, and challenges, creative, joy in discovering	*Instigator/dictator* Wants to control—often without participating, feels they have the right to be first in everything, irritable, destructive, impulsive, reckless, aggressive, difficulty with sharing and cooperation, ambivalent, uninterested, apathetic

	Balanced expressions	Imbalanced expressions
Physical expressions	Supple, springy, harmonious movements, flexible, good coordination and gross motor skills, controlled physical activity, desire for movement	Inhibited movements; stuck, delayed, or jerky movement patterns; poor gross motor skills; stiff and inflexible; reddened eyes, weak vision; tension and cramping in the head, neck, and shoulder area; tendency toward muscle cramps; dizziness with blood rushing to the head; abdominal pains
Wood Element developmental characteristics and expressions	Good visual and spatial perception; good orientation; distance of hands and body from objects; distance of bat from ball; catching objects; drawing and creating balanced images or objects, etc.; good judgment and foresight in planning of physical movements and later strategy and planning skills; decisive, confident, and assertive in actions	Poor spatial perception and low self-esteem; inhibitions toward movement; uncertain gait; motor and sensory development disturbances (particularly in the lower extremities); self-aggressions, e.g. nail-biting, hitting the head, legs, or other self-aggressive acts

All expressions listed in this chart will vary according to age and stage of development.

When observing the above chart, it is important to remember that children flow in and out of balanced and imbalanced expressions of each Element. One might even observe large shifts moment to moment as they watch young children playing. The moment-to-moment, day-to-day, and week-to-week shifts are the dance of Five Element growth as children try out new expressions and experience the responses of the environment around them. When children are struggling and showing signs of imbalanced behaviors of certain Elements, stop and look at the overall environment to see if some of the fundamental levels of elemental expressions are being hindered by the child displaying the behavioral difficulties. For example, if a child suddenly becomes aggressive and he does not typically have this kind of reaction, look and see if he is being allowed to move enough or express his creative ideas in the play situation. This is just one example of many possibilities from the Wood Element. The following list gives some general guidelines for areas to inquire about when a child is struggling in the development of some of the Wood Element expressions.

Questions for Observation
THE ENVIRONMENTAL SUPPORTS FOR WOOD ELEMENT DEVELOPMENT

1. Does the child have enough physical space and time in her life to jump, run, balance, swing, and discover large, playful movements?

2. Does the child have physical objects, items, or playmates in the environment (other than electronic toys or computers) that encourage imagination, creativity, and 3D discovery for self-initiated games and playing?

3. Does the child have space to be loud, shout, and use playful screaming and various verbal sounds that express outbursts of energy?

4. Does the child have large toys for building with—large blocks for stacking and building forts and walls, or large geometric-shaped pillows to build and climb on?

5. Does the child have access to age-appropriate opportunities that allow her to be creative and use planning skills and strategies?

EXPRESSIONS OF THE WOOD ELEMENT IN CHILDREN—KINDERGARTEN AND ELEMENTARY SCHOOL (5–7 YEARS OLD)

1. How does this child move and appear in their coordination for his age level?

2. How does the child approach craft or work projects—with original ideas or the need to copy another child's ideas?

3. Have there been any problems with eyesight?

4. Does this child like to participate in physical activities in school or have interest in sports outside of school?

5. Does the child get tired easily when doing physical activities?

6. What frustrates this child the most and how does he express it?

7. How assertive is this child in getting what he wants?

8. What is this child's self-confidence like?

9. How does the child express himself creatively?

10. Does this child bite his nails or show any signs of self-aggressive acts?

Developmental Requirements of the Early Expression of the Wood Element

1. Room and time to have large, expressive movements.

2. Examples of appropriate expressions of anger and guidance to express anger appropriately.

3. Mentoring and games that teach the self-awareness and observation of the four primary emotions of anger, sadness, fear, and happiness in others and the self.

4. Opportunities to make decisions and to be given choices whenever possible.

5. Opportunities to lead and follow with peers.

6. Opportunities to be creative—for example, make up games with different objects, color on blank pieces of paper, journal events in life through drawings, or build or create large and small objects with random supplies.

7. Room to shout and express loud noises.

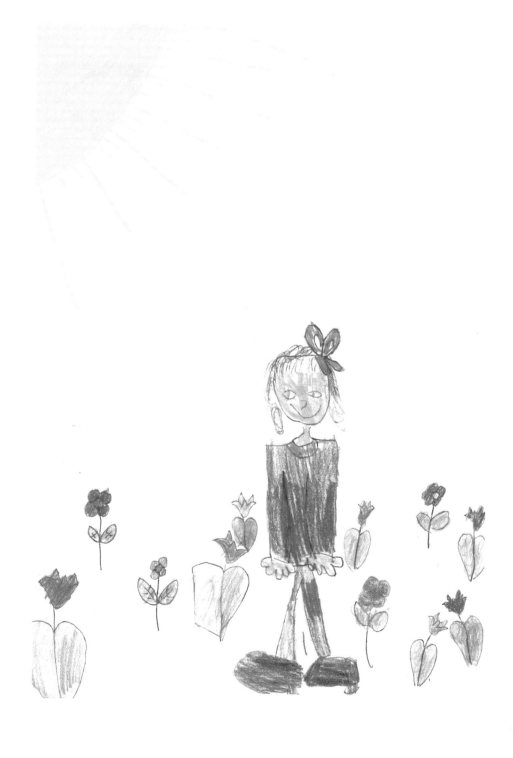

CHAPTER 5

The Fire Element in Child Development

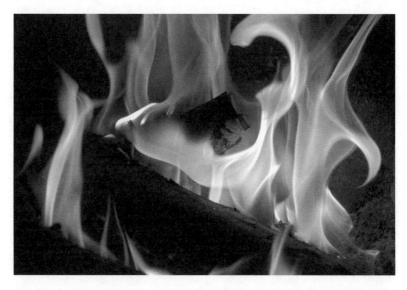

The Fire Element gives to us a vitality and enthusiasm for life. Japanese medicine says that the spirit of man lives in the heart like a silent guide, giving us the warmth for all aspects of relationships, communication, joy, and even sorrows in life. As in the previous chapter about the Wood Element, this chapter will begin with an experience. So, once again, open your imagination and read the following.

Adults
A Fire Element Experience

It is a beautiful summer day and you look out of your window to see the sun shining bright. A group of cyclists pass the window, riding through the town; the family next door is playing with their dog and going to the children's park; a couple dressed in beach attire are loading their car for a day of swimming at the lake. Everywhere you look, nature is buzzing with activity and there is an excitement in the air that feels full of energy. You gather your bags and feel your own vitality as you walk out the door to go to the market. Your steps feel energized with the warmth of the sun and gentle summer breeze, giving you a sense of lightness in your stride. In your first steps, you feel an open-heartedness that is ready to greet the world, and your eyes feel alive, like the nature around you. You notice the birds in the trees teaching their young to fly and hunt for food, as well as the bees gathering pollen and whispering messages to each other in the buzzing of their wings. The fruit-bearing trees, with their powerful trunks, have a particular radiance, energizing the whole scene. The warmth of the day seems to be giving everything the energy for activity and there is a sense of purposefulness and connection between everything in motion. You notice again that your heart feels a light openness in seeing the activity around you, and there is an awareness of an unspoken meaning in life that fills the moment. You pause for a moment to feel a warm joy through your whole body and take a deep refreshing breath, energizing your pace once again as you walk on.

As you continue your walk to the market, you hear classical music in the distance which you follow to find an open-air concert in a nearby park. You notice again a lighthearted and joyful energy in the air as you observe the mingling and seated crowd. The music is fitting for the summer day and its playful harmony influences the activity of the spectators. You find a seat toward the back where you can view the entire scene. Your eyes are drawn to the conductor, fascinated and spellbound by his orchestration. You ask yourself what it is that attracts your attention. You watch intently how he directs the whole scene with delicate movements, gestures, and expressive pauses. Again, you sense this deep, joyful feeling inside. Where does it come from?

A gentle lift of the arm, and the violins join in all together; a short confirming glance toward the flautist and she repeats her playful melody. Everything seems to be in perfect harmony, note for note, and mutually sustaining. Yes, that's it! A picture filled with symmetry, rapport, and unity of the orchestra working together. It is not just the music alone that evokes this feeling of joy; it is the connection of the whole orchestra following the inspiration of the conductor as he leads their collaborative performance with an ability to communicate what is needed with a glance or his whole body. His whimsical passion for the piece that is being played is apparent in his facial expressions, and the orchestra feeds off his enthusiasm and open-heartedness as he communicates his joy for the perfection of their harmony. As the piece ends, you feel touched by his presence, and how the individual musicians were affected by his presence and moved to add their own personal tone to the total composition.

A tearful sense of joy streams through you as you recognize how moved you are by the openness of the conductor in his animated performance that touched everyone in and observing the performance. A moment of awe and silence and then whistles and applause from the crowd show that most were moved in some way by the performance. You sit back to enjoy the rest of the concert as you recognize the contagious effect of allowing the lightness and joy of the heart to express itself to the world and others.

Expression of the Fire Element

The Fire Element gives us the capacity for joy and enthusiasm and the ability to express these. Tasks in work, relationships, and all areas of life require energy to be undertaken, and problems can be solved with vivacity when Fire is free to express itself in our lives. The term "twinkle in the eyes" takes on a deeper meaning when we look at the Fire Element. It is in the eyes that the vitality of life and an individual's Fire Element energy can be seen as it radiates out to or shields itself from the world.

The ability to clearly express our emotions and initiate closeness with others so that we can develop and maintain relationships comes to us in the development of the Fire Element. All forms of communication that create opening and connection with others are from a developed Fire Element capacity. Skillful verbal communication that allows others' opinions and invites others' ideas and voices is a Fire Element quality. The quality of warmth in other forms of human interaction and the energy that expresses passions in life come from the Fire Element. The mature development of Fire gives us the ability to have heartfelt interests in connecting with others and their circumstances. True companionship and friendship become possible as the Fire Element moves and unfolds within us. The emotional recognition of self and others develops in this Element and the ability to be with the emotional expressions of others.

Fire gives us the ability to have an openess in life, regardless of what struggles we encounter. This manifests in many ways. When faced with opposition and strong differences in discussions, Fire keeps our communication and heart open with a warmth and articulate nature that allows all voices to be heard. It is the keeper of the atmosphere so that all viewpoints can be heard in a group while still holding the purpose of the conversation in the foreground. Fire's clear, articulate sense of reality makes it easy for us to evaluate situations and give feedback that supports self-esteem. An inner knowing that it is important for all to be able to express their purpose in life comes from the Fire Element energy and gives the capacity for us to allow others' feelings to be felt and expressed.

A self-confident speaker has a well-developed Fire Element as it gives the capacity to express humor, wisdom, deep truths, and the lightness of life and all of its aspects. The Fire Element has a quality of radiation that touches others from the deepest of sorrows to the freeness of uninhibited joy. Truly, one of the primary gifts of Fire is a lightness of being that allows us to laugh at ourselves in our human nature, look on the bright side of life, and survive the many heartfelt struggles we experience in the world.

The chart below shows the Fire Element expressions and correspondences with nature. This information will allow you to begin to observe the environmental, physical, behavioral, and psychological expressions of each Element in life.

Correspondences and characteristics of the Fire Element

Season	Summer
Climate	Hot
Tissue/body parts	Blood vessels
Bodily fluids	Blood, sweat
Orifices	Ears
Sensory organs	Tongue
Sensory function	Speech
Taste	Bitter
External, physical form of expression	Complexion, face color
Balanced behavioral expressions	Communicative, intuitive, empathic, sensitive to others, optimistic, charismatic, enthusiastic, lighthearted, openness to all of life's experiences, ability to express warmth for self and others, ability to communicate humor appropriately
Behavioral expression under stress	Anxious, cold and detached, inappropriate humor, inability to hear what others are saying, misinterpretation of others' actions and communication, hypersensitivity, panicky, selfish, excitable, "Pollyanna," depression, poor memory
Balanced physical manifestation	Healthy complexion, good circulation, ability to sweat
Imbalanced physical manifestations	Heart palpitations, constant sweating, poor circulation, dizziness, pain in the chest, fatigue, red faced, inner restlessness, speech problems, raised shoulders, shock, pain in the solar plexus
Strength	Ability to experience and express sadness and pain
Verbal expression	Lively, expressive, laughing, giggling

Children
Expression of the Fire Element

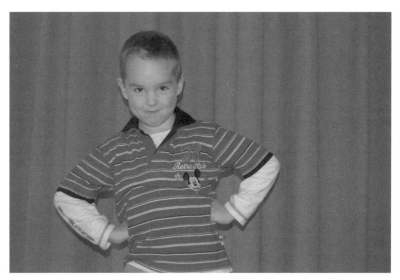

A child with balanced Fire Element energy will be noted for the enthusiastic and spontaneous way she presents different ideas for play. Her liveliness entices and motivates other children. She is sought after in group games because she quickly understands the importance of team cooperation and often supports weaker children. Because she accepts the weaknesses of others, they feel encouraged to show her their best side. As a playmate, she supports others with a self-assuredness of her own qualities and has the ability to keep them present without making the other children feel small or less than equal in the presence of her confidence. Since she is really happy, laughs heartily, and meets others with sensitivity and loving attentiveness, she is a favorite playmate who gladly accepts invitations and contributes to maintaining play relations.

Always interested in her surroundings, she shows no rejection toward children in the class who may be difficult or unmotivated by group activities. She is an especially good partner to children with these tendencies because of an innate sense of equality. A child with these Fire qualities focuses on the good in other children and not their weaknesses. Her inclusive way of communication expresses itself with warmth and sensitivity. She knows just how to be with other children in a way that opens doors to relating and connecting.

She is very good in situations where she must realistically estimate the progress or the effectiveness of a game. Since she radiates confidence, usually built on a sense of being appreciated and loved, she possesses a natural authority that the other children gravitate toward. Ingrained in this strong expression of the Fire Element is a form of wisdom that knows how to deal with conflicts in a group and does not instigate or provoke disturbing behavior.

When necessary, she expresses herself with clear, precise, and meaningful words, which is one of the diverse levels of communication that she always has at her disposal. Alert and interested eyes mark the strong expression of the Fire Element in a child, accompanied by a healthy complexion with light rosy cheeks and a liveliness that motivates others, even in quiet play.

Brigitte and Lani are 13 years old. A new boy, Johan, entered their middle school class from another school. During the break he was always sitting alone in the school yard while the other boys were playing soccer. In the beginning, the boys asked him if he would join them and he said no. He sat alone for a couple of weeks during the break. Brigitte and Lani decided to approach Johan and told him that if he didn't try at least once to play in the group with the boys, he wouldn't be able to make friends in the class. At first, he refused harshly, saying "I don't want to!" and wouldn't talk anymore. But they did not give up on him. They sat next to him and continued to talk. He understood that they were sincerely interested in him and he opened up. He confided that he thought he was not very good at soccer, and if he played with the boys, they would like him even less. Brigitte and Lani told him it was very important that he give it a try.

The girls then went to the two leaders of the group playing soccer, and asked them to invite Johan to play soccer so that he could be included and make friends with everyone. They did this in a compassionate and playful way so that the leaders listened to their request without feeling embarrassed or ashamed for not noticing that Johan was sitting by himself. The girls then also quietly whispered that Johan wanted to play but was afraid he wasn't good enough and that if he made a mistake they wouldn't like him. The boys took the cue as the girls asked them nicely to consider Johan was new and not laugh, joke, or ridicule him as they did with each other in their familiar ways when they played poorly.

When the boys asked Johan to play soccer again, he did. He was much better than he thought—and better than the other boys thought he would be. Since that afternoon, he was taken in as a new friend in the boys' group.

Imbalanced Expressions of the Fire Element

When Fire Element energy is disturbed, the liveliness and vitality of a child can be expressed in powerful and impulsive ways. The child will typically have bursts of short, unrestrained movement that resemble a wild horse just set free, which are driven from quick-arising reactions and a need to express oneself emotionally. These responses are often directly related to a situation, the environment, or beliefs that the environment is trying to contain their heart's desire in the moment, but with the lack of ability to coordinate and control the body movements. When these explosive expressions happen, they are accompanied by a red face and sweating which quickly leads to fatigue and exhaustion. When a child with imbalanced Fire energy is introduced to new adults or children, he often acts rudely and shows signs of mistrust.

A disposition of chronic unhappiness is another sign of Fire imbalance, leading to a constant search for distraction, diversion, and stimulation. This blocks the child's natural spontaneity of playfulness and lightness in imaginary games. This child is often bored in play situations and intolerant of activities that take place over a long period of time.

A child with imbalanced Fire Element expressions often has a quick understanding of the interactive dynamics of cooperative or academic games. She finds it difficult to wait for the instructions to be complete because she does not understand that it takes the other children longer to understand. She will have a burning desire to communicate her knowledge immediately, usually before the teacher has finished giving the instructions or explanation of the work. This child is often the one asking the teacher the question about the next step in math, before she has the chance to finish teaching the first. There will be an impatience with other children who do not understand as quickly. An inflated sense of self-confidence may cause this child to appear to be too much of a show-off, too arrogant, or too ambitious a playmate for weaker children.

Moods can change quickly from sky-high exuberance to intense sadness, and from hectic and restless to mentally absent and mute. This child can become consumed in excessively comparing and evaluating the most minute details, and can have strong reactions and emotional outbreaks. The child with imbalanced Fire Element expressions may also appear to be the eternal wisecracker or class clown, as the natural joyfulness of Fire struggles to find balanced ways to express humor.

Almost always behind this type of behavior in children with Fire imbalances is the appearance of a lack of awareness of other children's feelings, which also leads to feeling unappreciated by others when they do nice things for another child. A general lack of connection with others could be another visible trait, which leads to a child having inconsistent experiences of herself as she is rewarded for behaviors that appear to show consideration for others and punished for behaviors that appear inconsiderate or inappropriate. Without the depth of feeling connection for others, this inconsistency can be confusing for a child and create more reactions and outbursts. It also makes it difficult for a child to maintain friendships and relationships. Reactions from peers and adults in the environment, such as rejection or expulsion from games, produce a real basic anxiety in these children ("I am *not* OK!") and they withdraw further from social contact.

Disturbances in group settings with children with underdeveloped or imbalanced Fire Element tend to involve repeated inquiry about information—even when it is explained step by step, over and over again—which comes from a difficulty to slow down. Instructions from a parent or teacher are not heard because the child's mind is talking and communicating with him on the inside. He fails to hear all of the instructions because he has an anxious need to come to the end of the instructions and feels that he already understands what needs to be done. This is different from an inability to decipher the information with the other noises in the room, as in the Water Element imbalances which we will talk about later. Overall, a Fire Element imbalance in a child has the appearance of something running faster on the inside in the child's perceptions, driving him to react quickly or at his own internal pace. The child can feel out of sync, disconnected from the world and others, and frequently misunderstood.

The inability to speak clearly and meaningfully without rambling or stuttering is another conspicuous sign for Fire Element imbalances. When a child with Fire Element imbalances is sitting or painting, the observer notices raised shoulders and tensed arms, as well as cramped fingers. Illnesses often are expressed with high fevers and inflammation, or pain in the ears and neck.

Sebastian began stuttering from time to time when he was three years old. In the small, private preschool and kindergarten he attended, this was never a problem. He was always a happy and sunny child. His liveliness and vitality was infectious and influenced the whole class, and his presence was missed by all when he wasn't at school due to illness. He was very interested in the other children and had many friends. In particular his quickness in offering his opinions pleased the teachers.

This changed quickly after he entered elementary school at age seven. He started his new school full of joy and excitement. As the days went on, however, he found that all his efforts to enter into conversation with his new schoolmates ended in ridicule if he stuttered. He became quieter and quieter in school. When his excitement did arise and he tried to express it, his stammering was accompanied by blushing. The embarrassment of this created strong feelings of anxiety and his stuttering worsened dramatically. To avoid the danger of having to speak, he withdrew completely from the social circle of children in his class and could be seen sitting alone or reading a book at break times.

Now eight years old, he appears on the outside to be mentally absent and not interested in dealing with others, although his mother says he longs to have a friend. In class, when the teacher calls on him to speak, he perceives this as intimidation. He rarely participates verbally in lessons, even though he knows the material well. Simply imagining that he must say something in front of the entire class leaves him speechless. In this way, a happy child became a saddened and often depressed child.

Environmental Influences on the Development of the Fire Element

The Fire Element in a child arises and individuates out of the Back Family and *Keiraku* in early child development. Research shows that within the first 12 minutes of being out of the womb an infant is making attempts to communicate with her surroundings and will begin changing the sound of her cries and body movements to repeated acknowledgments from her parents or care-givers. Even though these early expressions are not yet specific to the undeveloped Fire Element in a child, this acceptance, mirroring, and invitation for the child to be in the world support the later individuated expressions of Fire in a child.

If a child grows up in an environment that accepts and engages with her innocent, impulsive reactions and responses to her daily life, she is offered a mirroring that invites the innate nature of the life *Ki* to express itself and expand in the world. Many people struggle with a sense of purpose in their life, and it is in the Fire Element that this spark and impetus to live fully and with a sense of purpose is born. A child needs to be engaged, played with, and seen as a meaningful human being to develop a confidence to express himself in life. A child described as having a "twinkle in his eye" is a child thought to be so mischievously spontaneous and full of energy that it often gets him into trouble with his impulsive nature and need to do what is fun and exciting in the moment. How that child's passionate nature to explore is dealt with will make a difference in how he will step into that innate nature to follow his need for lightness and passion in life.

A child who is encouraged and engaged in healthy verbal and physical relationships will develop an inner and outer sense of himself to stand up in the world and communicate what is important to him in his life. The opposite is also true: if a child is discouraged, berated, or met with sarcastic judgments about his actions and ideas in life, he will become insecure and unsure of himself and his self-meaning in life. This behavior can be seen in children who repeatedly get discouraged easily or are afraid of trying new things for fear of ridicule. They might even have a negative self-talk and judgmental voice that puts them down, telling them that they aren't good enough or that their thoughts are stupid. They lack the confidence to be spontaneous and fun.

In Fire, it is the caretaker's role to listen and watch for the early signs of communication in a baby and toddler, and to understand the innocence of their expressions and lack of intentionality. Verbal communication and self-awareness of feelings and emotions are a mature Fire Element expression. Young children in the early stages of their energetic development, meaning the Three Families and *Keiraku*, express their passion, enthusiasm, desires, feelings, and emotions without distinction or self-awareness of what they are expressing. How adults and other mentors interpret these expressions and support the full movement of the Element physically and verbally without judgment or shame will affect the Fire Element development in a child. Patient guidance, acceptance, lightheartedness, and joy in the early attempts to communicate strong desires and needs from children will support balanced development of the Fire Element later.

The ability to begin learning how to recognize the distinctions and verbally communicate all four of the primary emotions—anger, sadness, fear, and joy—is a sign of the readiness of a child to enter into the Fire Element stage of development. When children are encouraged to recognize their feelings, use emotional language, and problem-solve uncomfortable feelings and conflicts appropriately with others, they develop a healthy self-acceptance and awareness that nurtures a positive self-esteem and resiliency in life. When children develop self-confidence through self-acceptance, they naturally have an openness and acceptance of other children that allows for relationships, friendships, and connections on many levels of life.

Exercises
IS THE CHILD READY FOR FIRE ELEMENT DEVELOPMENT?

The *Keiraku* exercises used to assess the readiness of a child to begin focusing on the development of the Fire Element can be used for the Water or Fire Element assessments with a child. This is because the *Keiraku* are the representation of six energy pathways in the body that are a combination of the 12 meridians in an undifferentiated state. Two of the *Keiraku* for the Fire Element contain the combination of the undeveloped separate pathways of the Small Intestine and Bladder meridians, and the Heart and Kidney meridians. The following exercises are used to assess Fire Element readiness because of the strong emphasis on the arms, which is a Fire Element quality.

Movement Exercises
1. Wheelbarrow

Mark out a distance of three yards/meters. At the start line, one child decides to be the wheelbarrow and the other child decides to be the one that pushes the wheelbarrow. The wheelbarrow child goes on to all fours at the start line. Then the partner lifts up the child's legs. The wheelbarrow child stretches out their arms and their entire body. The image of a wheelbarrow helps the children to understand what they should be doing. To support the muscle tone in the back of the wheelbarrow child, a beanbag or something similar is placed on the back. This piece of "luggage" now has to be transported to the finish line. The partner child supports the legs of the wheelbarrow child as their arms are used to walk to the finish line.

QUESTIONS FOR ASSESSMENT

1. Is the wheelbarrow child able to walk the distance of three yards/meters?
2. Can the wheelbarrow child keep his back straight?
3. Can the wheelbarrow child keep his legs extended?

4. Can the wheelbarrow child keep his arms extended?

5. Does the wheelbarrow child rotate the pelvis while doing the movement?

2. Feeling/Mood Barometer

Prepare a few pictures or photos that show a person expressing different feelings or moods. Have a large mirror ready. The feelings/moods in the pictures should be evident from the body language, gestures, and facial expressions.

Now show the children one picture after another and ask them to imitate the feeling or mood.

QUESTIONS FOR ASSESSMENT

1. Does the child recognize the feeling/mood that is depicted?

2. Can the child imitate the feeling/mood?

3. Can the child name the feeling/mood?

4. Does the child know the feeling/mood well enough to express it without the aid of a mirror?

If you answered no to any of the questions in Movement Exercises 1 and 2, the following exercises can be done to help further the development of the *Keiraku* in a 5–7-year-old child.

Keiraku Development Exercises
1. Magic Spell

This exercise is suitable for a group of three or more children. It's fine for it to become animated and for there to be lots of laughter.

a. Tell the children that a mysterious spell is going to make them suddenly stick to each other and that only another spell can set them free again.

b. "You can move around the room any way you like—you can run, jump, hop on one leg, crawl, walk on your heels or on tiptoe, or any way you can think of. But pay attention—when the magic spell 'Foot magic!' is called out, two people must come together really fast, and follow the order of the spell to stick to each other with one or both feet. This can also include more than just two children."

c. Once all the children have found a partner and are moving around the room with one or both feet stuck together, the setting-free spell is called out: "One, two, three, and now you're free!" Everyone moves around the room freely again. Further spells could be for magic to stick together at the elbows, knees, head, bottom, and so on. Let the children have fun and be creative.

2. The Crabs Play Soccer

This exercise can be done with one child if the trainer/parent/ teacher/therapist joins in, or with a group. Here the *Keiraku* of the Bladder, Small Intestine, Kidney, and Heart meridians are involved. The exercise can therefore be used to stimulate the Water Element as well as the Fire Element.

a. The children are divided into two groups (or the trainer and one child play together).

b. The groups (or the trainer and child) take up positions by opposite walls of the room. In the middle of the room lies a ball. The objective of the game is for each group to reach the ball as fast as possible, going crab-wise—with hands and feet on the floor, knees bent at right angles, belly facing the ceiling, and bottom lifted up off the floor. Each group tries to shove the ball to the opponent's side. If a goal is scored by the ball touching the opponent's wall, everyone goes back to the starting position and the game is played again from the beginning.

3. Nicking Socks

This game is suitable for groups of at least six children. Each child needs to be wearing loose-fitting socks.

a. On command, everyone crawls around the room and tries to pull as many socks as they can off the other children's feet and stick them into their own waistband. This contest gives rise to much laughter and romping.

b. To calm the group down afterwards, all the socks can be put into a bag, and the child who collected the most socks is blindfolded and has to try to find the matching pairs. Can it be done?

4. A Sad Little King
This game is for three or more players.

a. "One of you plays the king, the others are his subjects. You, the subjects, try—one after the other—to make the king laugh. So you need a few ideas! For example, you can bring the king funny little presents and/or make faces. But most important is always to ask the king very politely: 'Would Your Majesty be so good as to accept this modest gift from an unworthy subject?'"

b. The person who manages to make the king laugh or smile can be the next king.

Overview
Expressions of the Fire Element in children

	Balanced expressions	Imbalanced expressions
Behavioral expressions	*Sunshine child* Assimilates thoughts and ideas, joyful, alert, enthusiastic, loving, optimistic, open-hearted, charismatic, devoted, inclusive of other children	*Prankster, class clown* Anxious, insensitive, restless, mistrustful, very moody, show-off behavior, difficulty gathering information from environment and assimilating thoughts and ideas

Physical expressions	Lively, rosy complexion, laughs a lot, happy, twinkling eyes, warm hands and feet, warm body, good circulation	Speech disorders (e.g. stuttering), poor circulation, red tip of the tongue, hunched shoulders, tense arms, cramped fingers, inflammation of ears and throat, sensitive reaction to slight drops in temperature, high fever, sleep disorders, inner restlessness, canker sores
Fire Element developmental characteristics and expressions	Communication of thoughts, feelings, and desires in many ways (e.g. body language), congruent with feelings, facial expressions, expressing warmth and passion through touch and speech	Inability to communicate thoughts or ideas clearly, rambling descriptions without making a point clear, impatient in communication

All expressions listed in this chart will vary according to age and stage of development.

Questions for Observation
THE ENVIRONMENTAL SUPPORTS FOR FIRE ELEMENT DEVELOPMENT

1. Is the child in environments that accept and allow him to express his feelings, ideas, and interests?

2. Is the child in environments that are warm and encourage self-expression without ridicule and sarcasm?

3. Is the child in environments that are joyful, light, playful, and appropriately spontaneous?

4. Does the child have room to verbally communicate his feelings, ideas, and warmth to others in his life, and is he given examples of this?

5. Does the child have the opportunity to express his personal humor and experience other forms of appropriate humor in his life?

6. What kind of communication is expressed in this child's daily environment?

7. What kinds of loving relationships are in the life of this child?

8. Does the child have the opportunity to develop playmates and friendships?

EXPRESSIONS OF THE FIRE ELEMENT IN CHILDREN—KINDERGARTEN AND ELEMENTARY SCHOOL (5–7 YEARS OLD)

1. How alert does this child's eyes look?

2. How does this child communicate her ideas, emotions, desires, needs, and enthusiasm?

3. What is the child's overall speech like?

4. How aware is the child of other children's feelings and weaknesses?

5. How well does the child follow directions and work in group activities in school?

6. Does this child have friends that she plays with and, if so, what do they do and what is their playing like?

7. How is this child valued by her classmates?

8. How does this child respond to other children who are displaying learning challenges?

9. How does the child respond to other children who are weaker or less skilled than her in group activities?

10. How does this child express humor and joy?

Developmental Requirements of the Early Expressions of the Fire Element

1. A warm, welcoming acceptance of the infant into the family's life.

2. Experience of laughter and lightheartedness in the environment and self.

3. Acceptance and understanding of all emotional expressions as valid and real in a child's early communication.

4. Encouragement to express oneself verbally and from the heart.

5. Warm and heartfelt communication from adults, siblings, and daycare environments.

6. Acceptance of feelings and emotions, and support in learning how to recognize and express them verbally.

7. A warm, loving environment and understanding of innocence in the process of learning to express feelings, desires, and enthusiasm.

8. Examples of open-hearted acceptance of others less fortunate.

9. Examples of clear verbal communication with emotions, disagreements, and conflicts.

10. Examples of healthy relationships and healthy relating to others in the world.

11. Room to play, be spontaneous, and have fun in life.

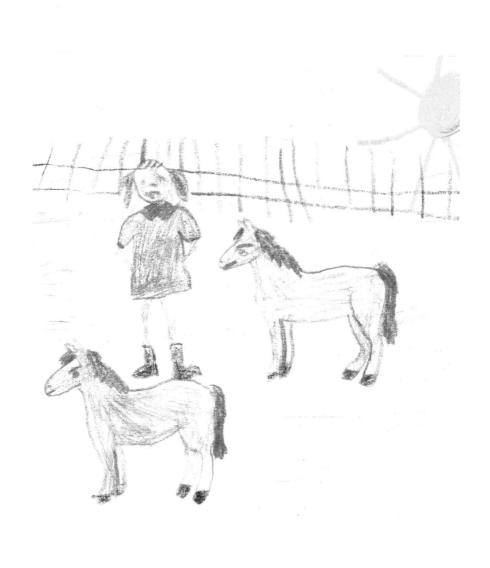

CHAPTER 6

The Earth Element in Child Development

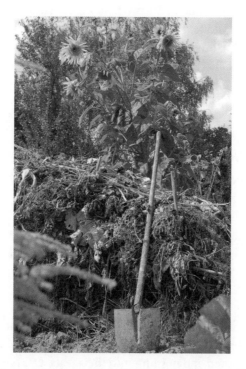

The Earth Element is the center of all the Elements. If we consider the analogy of the actual functions of the physical earth in our lives, we can see what this Element brings to us daily. We wake up and place our feet on the earth in the morning and we return to the same

support to rest at night. Our food, air, water—everything that
sustains us—come from and are created by the elements of this
planet that supports us. All of life as we consciously know it pivots
around this solid presence that humankind readily takes for granted.

The Earth Element brings us the same support in our lives. All
of the other Elements, like life on the planet, rely on the Earth
Element to ground the experiences of life in the body and provide
nutrition and sustenance. The Earth Element supports the whole
digestive system and rules the taste buds. Just as it digests food and
drink in our lives, it digests thoughts and events. It supports the
whole body/mind/spirit with its ability to make life full and rich
by grounding our experiences with logic and bringing us into our
personal awareness and center. When we are confidently rooted in
our perspective in life, there is room for compassion, understanding,
and patience for others, while still holding the ground of personal
opinions and values, all of which are emotional capacities that the
Earth Element offers us.

Adults

An Earth Element Experience

You are car-pooling a group of eight-year-olds to a theater to see
a performance by an African dance company. The children know
that there will be drumming involved and the possibility of some
audience participation. Finding your seats at the theater, the children
are excited with anticipation and are having a difficult time staying
seated.

The show begins with a solo drummer entering the stage and
playing a very slow, rhythmic beat. He moves in time with the pulse
of the drum, which now sounds as if it is carrying the rhythm of a
human heartbeat. You feel your body begin to relax and observe the
children captivated and nestling into their seats. Even the most easily
distracted and physically active children in the group are spellbound
and calm in the presence of the drummer.

He is dressed in earthy clothes of terracotta, golden brown, and rich soil colors. His skin is smudged with clay and his clothes have leaves and moss sewn into them. As he drums and moves rhythmically, you are drawn to his grounded presence and the sureness of his feet. Every part of his body moves from his center and appears connected to his feet and drum. He dances in circles, symbolically, filling the stage with a grounded beat, preparing the soil of the stage for what is to come.

The beat begins to change to a more excited tempo, with higher-pitched tones that seem to leap out of the drum. Dancers dressed in bright green shades move out on to the stage in awe and excitement, and a second drummer with faster moves and rhythms enters with them. They too appear to move from their center and leap upward as the drummers meet in the center of the stage in their ritual beat and dance. You can feel the excitement of the new energy as the dancers move freely in their bodies, stretching out to the corners of the stage like tree branches catching the sun, while others seem to portray women sowing fields with seeds.

Another drummer, dressed in red, enters the stage. The beat is even faster and he is followed by women carrying baskets filled with fruit, wine, and bread. The stage is full of an aliveness and vitality as the colors dance joyfully in exotic moves circling around the drummers. It looks like a festival of happy villagers dancing in the delight of the field's bounty, as the drummers appear to magically puppeteer the dancers' choreography.

Just as the dance reaches its highest exuberance of energy, all three drummers drum a hard, low bong that immediately moves the dancers in unison into a slower, more graceful movement. And then a fourth drummer enters the stage, carrying a more reflective rhythm that makes you feel like breathing deeply and relaxing deeper into your seat. He is followed by women dressed in autumn colors gracefully dancing and spreading fallen leaves from pouches in their garments. The whole stage moves like the autumn wind and breath of a newborn child, calmly, without labor, and naturally.

土

You realize now that the performance is a ritual of the seasons as a fifth drummer, dressed completely in black, enters the stage, moving solidly, slowly, and profoundly with each beat and step. The dancers who follow swirl around the stage, and then stop with each beat of the drummer in black, matching his profound moves and beat. The stage lighting becomes dark like the winter sky, and the dancers look like dark snowflakes in the night, finding a pause in unison to a hidden rhythm that mimics a deep, sounding heartbeat.

Four of the drummers and dancers slowly move outward in a circle around the first earthy drummer who leads the beat. They kneel down, facing outward, in a circle on the stage. The earth drummer is their center; his drumming leads their every move as they reach out with the sound to the audience as if calling them to feel the beat of the earth and then back towards the center to give homage to the sound of the drum. It gives a profound, grounded, secure, and grateful feeling in the center of your belly and you notice, by their gestures, that the children too are touched deeply.

After the performance, you notice the children's behavior seems to be more grounded and solid. Again, even the most easily distracted and physically active children seem to be more peaceful, calm, and focused as they listen to the instructions for the next part of the show that will involve audience participation.

Expression of the Earth Element

Many of you reading this book might be able to recognize the feeling of suddenly perceiving the ease and solid presence of a person, without that person uttering profound words or performing conspicuous deeds. She is simply there, peaceful and radiating a sense of contentment and security. Even the most hectic situations do not disturb this repose; she is like a cliff amidst the breakers. One can trust this person, for she keeps her word. She is the type of person who knows just how to wait until a situation ripens, and then acts with experience and reflection. In teamwork, she creates the

土

solid ground in which real consensus can grow. Because of her good ideas and great capacity for concentration, the work flows smoothly. When colleagues need information, she has often already gathered what is needed and shares it readily.

She gives space and audience for others' opinions, and finds conciliatory words to re-establish harmony in the group when new ideas conflict with what has already been presented. This is often done by constantly recalling the common ground and direction of the group.

The strong expression of the Earth Element in an individual will often make her the natural caretaker of an office. She would be the one who initiates the sending of flowers to a sick colleague and a card with the signatures of everyone on the team. She makes sure that there is something to drink and snack on at a team meeting, and that there is a comfortable place in the company for everyone to share and meet. Her own workplace is nicely arranged, perhaps with a steaming cup of tea on the table and some luxurious plants in the room.

The opposite picture of this, when Earth Element energy is in disharmony, could show up in a person with an out-of-proportion broad-mindedness and a wish to mother everyone. Someone with this imbalance might make herself indispensable everywhere and has the need for the constant presence of others. Should one wish to hear the latest office gossip, her desk is the right place to find it. On the one hand, this person is excessively helpful and selfless but, on the other hand, woe to her colleagues if they once forget her birthday!

Correspondences and characteristics of the Earth Element

Season	Indian Summer/Late Summer
Climate	Humid
Tissue/body parts	Connective tissue, fatty tissue
Bodily fluids	Digestive juices
Orifices	Mouth, pharynx
Sensory organs	Mouth
Sensory function	Taste
Taste	Sweet
External, physical form of expression	Lips
Balanced behavioral expressions	Sympathy, compassion, readiness to help others, logical thinking, good memory, an ability to focus and concentrate, an ability to hold individual ideas and viewpoints, stable, receptive, ability to analyze and process information, feeling secure
Behavioral expressions under stress	Scattered thinking, over-accommodating, can't hold individual ideas or opinions, takes on characteristics of others and the environment, lack of independent thinking and ideas, difficulty with memory and concentration, over-zealous, meddlesome, over-thinking, worry
Balanced physical expressions	Firm, well circulated, resilient tone to muscles; balanced appetite; moist, healthy lips; good digestive system; good physical balance
Imbalanced physical expressions	Tiredness; fatigue; loose and flabby, or lumpy, fatty, and congested flesh; menstruation problems; varicose veins; dry or sticky mouth; inability to taste; problems with gums; digestive disturbances; overweight; colitis; irritable bowel syndrome; gas; bloating; ulcers

Strength	Persistence, grounded
Emotion	Compassion
Verbal expression	Singing

Children
Expression of the Earth Element

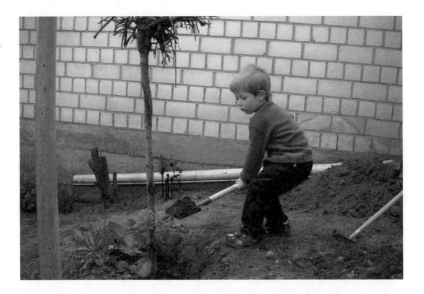

A child with a strong and balanced Earth Element energy is an enriching presence for any group. He is centered in his behavior and demeanor, without acting like a know-it-all. His secure sense of self-embodiment, view, and opinion of his environment gives him the ability to analyze and process information around him clearly. This centered knowing of self allows him to be open to advice and ideas from others. Without the advice from others, or a need to look for examples, his opinions in life come naturally, without seeking external confirmation from peers or adults. A child with a balanced Earth Element does not need to be the center of attention or make his opinions known; instead, he logically comes to his own conclusions without imposing the viewpoint on others. Because of

土

this undemanding style, other children and even adults feel drawn to this child. In sports, he has a steadfast and consistent nature in his demeanor and energy level. He is often the child who stays in for the whole game with a focused intention; he can be relied upon for his endurance and ability to keep playing without giving up.

This child will also show an everlasting readiness to help and support children or adults in need, and can accept help from others when required. In this way, his example strengthens other children who would not normally be inclined to offer assistance to others in need. When beginning a project in class, he makes sure that he has sufficient materials and tools to work with, but he does not claim the best or most beautiful for himself. This easy approach readily gets him what is desired.

Friendships are formed neither swiftly nor lightly. Yet, fundamentally, a child with a strong Earth Element characteristically approaches new friendships with an open-mindedness and readiness to help. A child with this nature often forms friendships with visibly less attractive children, but he knows and recognizes their qualities and promotes these so that, with the strengthening of their abilities, these children become attractive and sought-after friends. Towards close friends, this child is true and loyal in crisis situations. He can be counted on for unconditional acceptance and support in all situations in life.

When a child with a strong Earth Element is in a group, his presence and way of being creates a true group spirit. Such a group would be distinguished by behaviors that recognize the different strengths of individual group members and are considerate of the weaker ones. Strong Earth Element children create connections between opposites or those who are different. They can comfort or offer consolation, without insisting that it be accepted. The result is that all in the group feel a sense of a common ground and are able to contribute to group activities.

The Earth child feels fundamentally accepted and is content with self and the world. He is at home within himself and seeks out people and places that confirm this feeling and allow it to grow without calling it into question. A child with a strong Earth Element can endure unclear and uncertain times, knowing and trusting in an outcome that will restore peace. He can also—within a childlike framework—summon up patience. He can take in experiences and events and process them so that they become knowledge to be called on later when needed in other complex situations.

His capacity for abstraction and interpretation help him to apply experiences and events to other areas of life. He thinks logically and in an orderly way. He can concentrate well and is able to assimilate both familiar and foreign sensations and experiences. He is capable of integrating and processing these and recognizing different connections in life. He can be clingy and likes tickling, and shows a need for bodily contact, which he will seek out himself. At the same time, this child can offer closeness and warmth, both verbally and physically. Other children are very attracted to these qualities and feel very well taken care of with an Earth child. The following is an example of balanced Earth Element expressions in a child.

Charlotte was known in her class to be the teacher's helper. The other children looked up to her and often asked her for help when they didn't understand the directions given because she could explain to them what was needed without ridicule or arrogance. Every year, all the children in the fifth grade class took part in a Shakespearean play. This was a big deal because the children memorized their lines and auditioned for the different parts. There was an excitement in the class and even some jealousy between classmates who wanted the same roles. The teacher asked each child individually to leave the room to audition for their part, and a buzz of noise and excited squeals would fill the room as each child left and the previous one re-entered.

The supporting teacher supervising the classroom during the auditions later reported her observations of Charlotte in the class during the audition process. She was very moved as she watched Charlotte stay calm and reposed between each exiting and re-entering child, and then watched numerous children go to Charlotte and ask her to help them with rehearsing their lines

⊥

before their audition. One teary-eyed child after her audition even went to Charlotte for a comforting hug, and Charlotte assured her classmate that she would get a part in the play because the play would have all of them in it. Charlotte even asked during the auditions if they could all have a snack and something to drink to help them focus and calm down.

After the auditions and during the classroom discussion of what would happen next, it was Charlotte who asked thoughtful and reassuring questions about everyone getting a part in the play. Charlotte's unassuming and humble role in the classroom process was brought to the attention of the teacher, and out of this a special role was created. Charlotte was given the job of director's assistant and was even awarded a certificate at the end of the play for her compassionate and supportive role in helping all of her classmates and teachers with whatever was needed. Her focused, solid, and steadfast nature was felt by everyone in the play, and she humbly took the certificate at the end of the last performance and went back to her seat without showing off her well-deserved recognition.

Imbalanced Expressions of the Earth Element

A child with imbalanced Earth Element expressions uses this same collection of knowledge, impressions, events, and experiences to create his own reality. He ranks experiences one after another without the capacity to make connections between them and has difficulty focusing. In this way, his world remains incomprehensible and unsettling. He rejects everything strange, since it confuses his small reality still further. So, in his search for certainties, he is always dependent on others. This imbalance leaves a child constantly looking for recognition and affection. It is challenging for a child with Earth Element imbalances to experience and know his own feelings, which can lead to argumentative and opinionated behavior or constant complaining about a physical symptom. In this way, he is able to get individual attention that gives him some identity apart from other children.

A child with Earth Element imbalances can appear uncomfortable and ill-tempered, has quick-changing moods, and is often an unhappy, difficult-to-please comrade. He is filled with a striving to be recognized, secure, embraced, and wanted. Over-compensating devotion to others and a "helper syndrome" are common characteristics that leave others with the feeling of unclear intentions behind the behavior. This can be accompanied by exaggerated complimenting of others or overly-cuddly and ingratiating behavior which are an attempt to create self-recognition.

Another pattern that can arise in children with Earth Element imbalances is the tendency for the child to create self-rewarding systems with sweets after working. This behavior arises with children who need constant rewards after each step of accomplishment.

Frequently, the child with disturbed Earth Element energy feels overlooked, ignored, or passed over when decisions are being made. Then he feels sorry for himself, swallows his emotions, and withdraws; he may become internally restless and fidgety, which is soon externally visible. Since his sense of self is low, he often lacks the desire to do anything by himself, because playing by oneself requires self-worth and acceptance. The lack of groundedness and self-assuredness leads to excessive worrying in a child with this level of Earth imbalance. A child with this behavior will play the same situation over and over again in his mind or in conversation, finding it difficult to move on to the next activity or opportunity in a classroom or friendship.

A child with imbalanced Earth Element energy often develops repetitive motions—for example, tapping a pencil for a long time, rocking a chair on two of its legs instead of four, or doodling on a piece of paper. The behavior is like a scratched CD that can't move on and repeats itself in the same place over and over again. Regardless of how many times the child is instructed to stop a behavior, he will come back to it, forgetting he has ever been corrected.

Interruption of any daily routine creates anxiety in Earth-imbalanced children. Therefore, consistency in the living environment is important for this child. It is also important not to promise more than you might be able to honor. This child needs to feel he can rely

土

on what is promised as if his ability to stand is dependent on this. The feeling of common ground and the certainty of getting support are of great help to this child. Since he is often unable to organize his thoughts, he lacks a capacity to focus and then to proceed with the task. For that reason he is often concerned with things that other children have no problem looking over and arranging.

It is hard for a child with unbalanced Earth Element energy to live through transitions, to complete the step from one phase of life into the next. So he might still sit painting while others are already cutting, or he'll begin cutting even if he hasn't gotten that far in the exercise yet. This transitional disturbance can be expressed in problems with sleep, concentration, and eating. Physically, it can manifest itself as over-plumpness or extra fat. Clumsiness and uncertainty accompany weaknesses in the muscles and muscle tone in an Earth-imbalanced child. This child gets many bumps and bruises and tends to stumble over his own feet or fall from a chair.

Frequent hypochondriac behavior is also a possibility, in order to attract attention. Symptoms of sickness are stomach sensitivity accompanied by frequently inflamed corners of the mouth, diabetes, and inflammation in the area of the sinus cavities, jawbone, and gum tissues in the mouth or maxillary region. Eating disorders can range from a refusal to eat to overeating or the lack of ability to feel hunger or fullness in the stomach. For this child, a quiet and cheerful atmosphere at mealtime is a big help.

Moritz, age six, is a so-called "difficult eater." He picks at his food listlessly and finds fault with everything. When he comes back home from kindergarten at midday, he cannot sit at the table with his brother, but instead lets out all of his tension, during which his backpack flies in one direction, his shoes in another, and he picks a quarrel with his brother and mother. Once this "ritual" is over with, he sits down at the table. If his brother gets food before him or has his portion cut up into little pieces first, Moritz refuses his food.

From conversations with the mother, it becomes clear that the family does not have meals together and share their experiences and activities from the day. Since mealtimes with Moritz have become more and more difficult, no one in the family wants to sit with him at the table. In her despair, the mother now permits Moritz to eat in front of the television. At such times, he crams his food in without comment, without even registering what he eats.

In kindergarten, he stays with activities for only a short period of time, even the ones he has chosen himself. He is full of enthusiasm at first, but then his attention and endurance fail him. He runs to and fro and is always starting something new. When he wants something or needs help, it must happen right away; he cannot wait his turn. He is not satisfied with a short explanation or a request to wait a moment. Because of this, he is often rejected by the other children in group games.

In tense and unfamiliar situations, or in times of transition and change, Moritz reacts with a stomach ache, regardless of whether he is at home or in kindergarten. Conspicuously, he participates in rhythmic movement games with joy and complete concentration in school, where he has been seen as having more contact with himself and being more centered in his experience without the need for approval from others.

Environmental Influences on the Development of the Earth Element

As described in Chapter 1, the Earth Element belongs to the Front Family, which has to do with a baby coming into a sense of self. At the beginning, a newborn does not distinguish between self and other, and exists in what modern psychology calls a symbiotic state. The child feels hunger, moves and cries in response to the discomfort, and is fed and held if in a nurturing environment. This undifferentiated state of having needs met is, in an infant, one of the elemental foundations for bonding and a sense of trust in the world. Therefore, a nurturing environment that is attentive to the subtle needs of an infant and responds to cues lays the foundation for the later development of the differentiated Earth Element in a child.

As the nervous system of an infant continues to develop from multiple levels of stimulus in the environment through touch, sound, nutrition, rest, and holding, a child begins to discriminate self from the environment as her sight develops and she can see the distinction between self and others. When support of the child's individual needs occurs, a grounded sense of self can develop. Therefore, attentive and attuned caretaking is supportive for a child to come into a sense of self and her knowing of herself to be the center of her awareness. From this elementary central point of awareness, a child can interact and experience the other stimuli in the environment, and, as her needs continue to be met, a deep sense of contentment and trust in self can develop.

On the other hand, when an infant or child experiences stressful environments that have an effect on the nervous system, a child becomes over-attentive to the outer environment, not allowing a sense of self to be established in the foundational ground of initial self-awareness. The self-awareness that is developing experiences a lack of needs being met, a lack of satisfaction and contentment, and a sense of self not getting enough or being enough to get what is needed. Trust in the environment and the foundation of experience in life is unstable and inconsistent, making the integration of all of the experiences difficult to achieve. Therefore, safety, security, nurturing touch and holding, sufficient nutrition, responsiveness to infant needs, and peaceful environments with enough rest to be in contact with the world are important foundations for the later development of balanced Earth Element expressions in a child.

Exercises
IS THE CHILD READY FOR EARTH ELEMENT DEVELOPMENT?

The *Keiraku* exercises used to assess whether a child is ready to begin focusing on the development of the Earth Element can be also used for Metal Element assessments. The *Keirakus* for the Earth Element contain a combination of the undeveloped separate meridians of Metal and Earth—the Stomach and Large Intestine and Spleen and

Lung pathways. The following exercises are used to assess Earth Element readiness because of their strong emphasis on balance and nurturing, both of which are Earth Element qualities.

Movement Exercises
1. Standing on One Leg

"Put your right hand on your left shoulder and your left hand on your right shoulder. Now lift one knee, so that your leg can dangle freely and you're standing only on one leg." Then count to ten. Can the child manage to stand that long on one leg? Do the same on the other leg.

Second time round, the exercise can be done with eyes closed.

QUESTIONS FOR ASSESSMENT

1. Is the child able to stand like this for the count of ten?

2. Is one leg hanging freely, or is it leaning against the standing leg for support?

3. Does the child stand on one leg without wobbling?

4. Can she do the exercise equally well on each leg?

5. Do the hands stay on the shoulders?

6. Is the child also able to do the exercise with eyes closed?

2. Hopping

Have the child hop on one leg.

QUESTIONS FOR ASSESSMENT

1. Can he hop five times, one after the other, on this leg?

2. Can he do it on the other leg as well?

If you answered no to any of the questions from Movement Exercises 1 and 2, the following exercises can be done to help further the development of the *Keiraku* in a 5–7-year-old child.

土

Keiraku Development Exercises
1. Tree Nursery
This exercise is for a group of children.

   a. One child is the gardener, the others are the trees. All the trees get a hoop on the floor.

   b. The children stand on one leg inside their hoops—resting the bent leg against the calf of the other leg is allowed. The palms of the hands are brought together over the head. The gardener walks past the trees and asks them what they need—water, perhaps, or the soil may need to be loosened. Each tree can choose what it needs in order to thrive. However, when the gardener shouts "Break time!" the trees quickly leave their hoops and everyone, including the gardener, tries to get inside a different hoop. The child left without a hoop is the next to play the gardener.

2. Sometimes I'm Strong, and Sometimes I'm Weak
The child sits on the front edge of their chair.

Say to the child: "Lean forward so that your body is resting on your thighs, and let your arms hang at your sides. Let your head hang down in front as well, quite loose. Now, as you breathe in, you sit up slowly and grow up really tall. Stretch your arms out by your sides, with your palms facing forwards and your hands wide open. Raise the tips of your toes and press your heels firmly into the ground. As you breathe out, lean over forwards again and put your feet flat on the ground."

3. Snake Dance

   a. Tie together several ropes of varying thickness and lay them in wide curves on the floor. Now the children can balance barefoot on the ropes like a balancing beam.

   b. Next have them try to do it with their eyes closed. Can they do it?

c. And now the big challenge! One child holds on to the balancing child lightly from behind, while the latter, against this resistance of the leading child, attempts to make their way along the rope.

4. Nimble Feet

a. Everyone sits on a chair in a circle, with a piece of string about two feet long on the ground in front of them.

b. "When I say 'Go!' try to tie a knot in the string with your bare feet. Who'll be first, I wonder?"

5. Japanese Sedan Chair

a. Set up starting and finishing lines. The distance between is divided into three zones of equal length.

b. The children go to the starting line in groups of three.

c. Two players hold each other's hands to make the "sedan chair," and the third child gets into it. Now each team tries to cross the first zone as fast as possible—here they change roles. At the end of the second zone, they change roles again. Can the team make it as far as the finish line?

土

Overview

Expressions of the Earth Element in children

	Balanced expressions	Imbalanced expressions
Behavioral expressions	*The helper* Affectionate, likes snuggling, seeks out physical contact, open-minded, readiness to help others, at ease with self and the world, self-confident	*The meddler* Scattered thinking, difficulty in making casual connections and friends, uncertain, self-pitying, seeks affirmation and affection, complaining, worrying, meddlesome, helping when not needed, overbearing, attached, overly self-sacrificing
Physical expressions	Healthy, toned body, round features, balanced movement, good digestive system	Chronic gastrointestinal disorders, upper abdominal pains, dry lips, weak connective tissue, hard or overly flaccid tonicity of the body, clumsy, unbalanced, sticky saliva and sweat, sore or bleeding gums, inflammation around the mouth, diabetes, bruises easily, excessive appetite, no appetite
Earth Element developmental characteristics and expressions	Ability to focus and concentrate, ability to hold individual ideas and viewpoints, physical and mental balance	Hypochondria, inability to take thoughts full circle, over-thinking, worrying

All expressions listed in this chart will vary according to age and stage of development.

Questions for Observation
THE ENVIRONMENTAL SUPPORTS FOR EARTH ELEMENT DEVELOPMENT

1. What is consistent in this child's life?

2. Is the child in the same house he was born in or has he moved a number of times?

3. What changes have occurred recently in this child's life—for example, his bedroom in the house, new school setting, new friends, new babysitter, new sibling, new parent, or loss of a parent?

4. How does security show up in this child's life?

5. What are the child's eating habits like? Does he have a daily routine for eating? Does he have enough time to sit, eat, and digest his meals without interruption?

6. How consistent is this child's daily routine?

7. What kind of caretaking play space is set up for this child—for example, doll house corner, play kitchen, pet center?

8. What are the nurturing opportunities for this child—for example, gardening, baking, cooking with the family, pets?

EXPRESSIONS OF THE EARTH ELEMENT IN CHILDREN—KINDERGARTEN AND ELEMENTARY SCHOOL (5–7 YEARS OLD)

1. What is this child's concentration like?

2. When the class is playing, does the child hold the focus with the group or does she leave and get interested in something else?

3. How does this child react when asked for help or when support is needed from another child, teacher, or parent?

4. Does this child like to play alone sometimes?

土

5. What is this child's appetite and digestion like? Does she have any acidic or nervous stomach issues?

6. What is this child's center of gravity like? How balanced does she appear? Is she clumsy and awkward?

7. Does this child like gardening, digging in the dirt, making mud-pies, or playing with dough or clay?

8. Can the child feel something under her feet when stepping on it, and can she tell the difference between the objects she is stepping on?

9. Can this child follow instructions in the order given?

10. Does this child have her own thoughts, feelings, and opinions, and how does she respond to the thoughts, feelings, and opinions of others?

11. Does this child play nurturing games with stuffed animals, dolls, or other objects?

12. How does this child respond to change and transitions in life—for example, changing grades, the end of the school year, friends who move, changes in the house or family life?

13. How centered and self-aware does this child appear to be?

14. Does this child have a tendency to worry and repeat the same questions over and over again?

15. How does this child show compassion and awareness of others' needs?

Developmental Requirements of the Early Expression of the Earth Element

1. Healthy bonding with the primary caregiver.

2. Attentive caretaking that responds to the needs of an infant and child.

土

3. A nurturing home environment that allows room for rest, quiet, safety, security, consistency, and healthy nutrition.

4. Opportunities to nurture through play, pets, or gardening.

5. Consistent eating schedules and rituals without TV, books, or distractions other than sharing with family and friends.

6. Examples of helping others and group activity opportunities.

7. Support for individual ideas, feelings, and opinions.

土

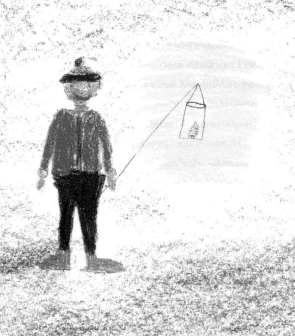

CHAPTER 7

The Metal Element in Child Development

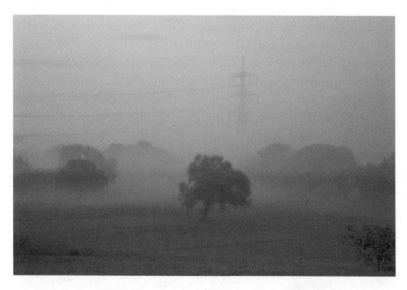

Of all the Elements, the Metal Element expresses the greatest degree of opposites when in balance. It brings into our lives the strength and precision of steel and a surrendering of permeability. The balance of our body, mind, and spirit is dependent on our ability to express both of these variables.

Metals in our community are precious. They are taken from the earth and transformed into tools for measurement, steel beams for skyscrapers, science and medical supplies, conductors for electricity, and national currencies. Wars have been fought and new lands have been sought for centuries for the discovery of the precious metal called gold. It is a substance that transforms from one shape to another without losing its original composition, and science today continues to make new discoveries with its uses. Metals create precise form, protection, structure, and value.

Likewise, the Metal Element gives us the capacity to assign value in our lives and to create our personal beliefs and structures. It can give us razor-sharp distinctions that help to define and create our personal boundaries. At the same time, its very nature is to transform and take on new shapes and structures when needed. Therefore, the Metal Element also gives us the ability to let go of old structures and beliefs and let in the new.

The Metal Element rules the skin, the primary sensory organ that gives us our first perceptions of the world and continues to define our environment and surroundings throughout our whole life. It is our container, interpreter, and communicator, as it helps to define our personal boundaries, interpret the outside world to our inner world, and then communicate it out again through touch and contact.

The lungs are also associated with the Metal Element. Together with the skin, they connect us to the outside world and the universe. The lungs create a rhythm and pattern in life that is predictable, which allows us to experience a sense of order, continuity, and belonging to everything. With each breath, we take in new air and let go of what is no longer needed. Our breath connects us to all living beings as we share the air with plants, animals, water, sky, and every nation in the world. From this arises a deep respect for and honoring of all life.

The Metal Element offers us the ability to discern differences without creating hard, cold judgments. To be open and acknowledging in life, while still holding personal boundaries, is a capacity of Metal—to live within our own belief systems, while honoring and acknowledging other ways; to let go of old structures, so that there is a possibility for the new to be born. The Metal Element is the alchemist, constantly in the process of transforming experiences into valuable information to serve all life.

Adults

A Metal Element Experience

The whisper of the steam engine and the grating of the steel brakes remind you of the punctuality of the train on which your close friend will soon be leaving. A long, quiet hug brings back to both of you once more the shared time, the happiness you had with each other, but also the discomfort of saying farewell. As you watch your friend climb aboard and find a window seat, the train slowly pulls out, and you feel a deep awareness of the final departure.

Leaving the station, the cold autumn wind blows in your face. A thought passes through your head: "How many departures and encounters occur day after day in this place?" It seems odd to you that this cold, steely building has sufficient room for so many deep experiences. Yet even your "steel thoughts" melt away at the sight of a mother with her newborn, saying goodbye to an older woman with tears in her eyes, while not far from you two lovers greet each other passionately. The walls of this building seem to symbolize a structure that allows a space of acceptance, and all these experiences find expression within these walls.

On your way back home, you look at slender, bare branches of the trees, which together with the swirling leaves are signs of winter coming. The leaves that still cling to the branches seem to attract the wind, as they dance together with the drifting dried ones it carries. Gleaming colors of shining gold, orange, red, yellow, and green show the respective degree of their change and make the process of separation of the leaves from the tree visible. When the time has come, the trees will be entirely bare and ready for the snow. You reflect on the analogy of what it takes to make the final changes in our lives when we are ready to take the next step toward something new. In every moment, nature expresses life and accepts all the changes that she brings with it. So you perceive a wisdom that nature demonstrates to you in simple things. You feel a deep sensation of recognition towards it.

Back home again, you open the door and glance once more over your shoulder. A great respect fills you, and you feel deeply connected with nature and its changing seasons, as well as with your friends, family, and all of humanity.

Expression of the Metal Element

When Sarah is in balance, she is an extremely self-disciplined individual. Her friends comment and joke with her all the time that she is naturally so perfect. She never has a bad hair day and her clothing is always coordinated and neat; even when she is walking out of the gym, where she goes regularly, her sweaty appearance and few misplaced hairs look perfectly planned. When going out to eat, she eats a perfectly balanced meal and doesn't even glance at the dessert tray. Something within her just knows right from wrong, good from bad, and how to stay within a regimen effortlessly without any doubt.

This woman lives by a schedule and strict routine. Punctuality is her middle name, and her friends feel a slight twinge of guilt in her presence because of her rightful presence and way of being. If they are running late, they can't help but apologize profusely and lament at how she is never late to any of their functions. Despite her own nature, she rarely passes judgment or has harsh words for those around her who have more difficulty with their schedules. She can't help but comment on what excites her: the new information about how good raw foods are for you, the healthy effects of walking 20 minutes a day, or the new iPhone reminder application and alarm that she just set up so she can give herself reminders. Finding the right way of taking care of herself and even the environment and world around her is her second nature. Showing up as a responsible individual in the world excites her, and she shares her interests openly.

At work, Sarah is known for being the rule keeper. She lacks a sense of humor when others joke about the boss, call in sick for a free day off, or leave work early. She has a deep respect for those in authority and the contract of her employment. Because of her natural inclination to honor rules and regulations, her employers use her as a confidential ear and her skills as a relay messenger to other employees about policy changes. It doesn't take long for her to get promoted to managerial positions. She has a keen sense of the boundaries existing between the management and employees, and is able to carry the ethos of the company out to those for whom she is responsible.

Sarah appears to be a confident, reflective person. She has an innate sense of self-worth that gives her a way of being that people naturally respect. Her friends admire her and at the same time are very aware of her boundaries. In her sense of rightness, there is also a sword-like ability that is sharp and clear. Her words cut right to the truth when someone is lying or not taking responsibility for their own wrong actions. Moments like these stop the breath in a room. If the person is quick to apologize or takes responsibility for the wrongdoing, Sarah is capable of acknowledging their strength and accepts them for their humanity, while still setting the consequences fairly. If they falter and continue to deny the conflict at hand, she is quick to let go of an employee or set a boundary for future communication until the issue is resolved. She can do this without remorse and with an attitude of exactness and non-judgmental consequences.

When Sarah is out of balance, life looks very different. She has a cold, bitter appearance and unforgiving energy that makes others feel like hiding when she walks in the room. "Hypercritical mode" is what she calls it when she recognizes she is in an unpleasant mood. Nothing is right because her perfectionist view of how to live and be in the world judges everything around her.

Her natural sense of order seems on hold, and simple decisions are laborious. Conflicts, tardy friends, and differing opinions are all reproached with an "above them all" attitude and self-righteous reprimand. Her self-discipline takes on a very hard, self-judging energy that is unforgiving and harsh. This she only shows to friends who are allowed to be close enough in her weaker, low-self-esteem moments.

Correspondences and characteristics of the Metal Element

Season	Autumn
Climate	Dry
Tissue/body parts	Skin, mucous membranes
Bodily fluids	Mucus
Orifices	Nose
Sensory organs	Nose
Sensory function	Smell
Taste	Sharp, spicy, astringent
External, physical form of expression	Skin, body hair
Balanced behavioral expressions	Ability to discern, define, create structure and order, analyze, be systematic, organized, orderly, neat, precise, self-disciplined, respectful, acknowledging, honoring, accepting; ability to assign value; ability to form strong but flexible belief systems; sense of the connection of self and all existence in the universe; sense of self-worth; ability to pace oneself; knows self-limits
Behavioral expressions under stress	Self-righteous, opinionated, hypercritical, disorderly and sloppy, dogmatic, perfectionist, prejudiced and judgmental, curt, lack of self-discipline, difficulty with authority, dogmatic, authoritarian, lack of self-worth, feeling isolated with an inability to connect, feeling alienated, inability to grieve
Balanced physical expressions	Strong cardiovascular and respiratory system; smooth and clear skin; balanced elimination; strong, lean muscles; good overall rhythm of body movements and organ functions

Imbalanced physical expressions	Asthma, respiratory infections and problems, allergies, irregular bowels, constipation, dry skin, sinus infections and headaches, dry cough, loss of smell, quiet or weak voice, easily susceptible to colds and viruses, cold hands and feet, skin rashes
Strength	Capacity to cough (getting rid of and letting go of what is no longer needed in life)
Emotion	Grief
Verbal expression	Metallic, nasal, whining, weepy voice

Children
Expression of the Metal Element

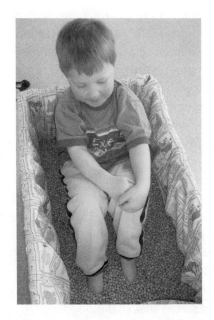

We recognize children with strong Metal Element characteristics most easily in situations when order, duty, fairness, and honor are in question.

A child with strong Metal Element expressions willingly allows himself to be guided by firm rules and exactitude in statements. For example, board games and games with rules are play activities that this child looks for and enjoys sharing with others. Structure and definition are needed to support this child's internal desire for quality in himself and his environment. They give them a sense of boundaries to learn and grow in.

When tasks are given out, this child is enthusiastic and thorough. He can, however, also recognize clearly when he is being taken advantage of and he then distances himself or refuses to participate. He has a keen sense of personal boundaries and is able to define and take the right amount of space needed while still being able to give intuitively what space other playmates need in their activities. An order and structure arises naturally in the playing space of a Metal Element child, allowing room for others to find their own place.

A child with strong Metal Element influence is very apparent in group settings when the leaders do not have everything laid out in perfect order. This child's tendency is to attempt to quickly create rules to get a feeling of some order or boundaries. This usually happens in inappropriate ways since this level of social skill is not yet developed in children and questioning authority is not accepted in most school settings. In these situations, a child might act out in whatever way will bring him most quickly to a disciplinary boundary, therefore giving him the sense of some order or container to be in, even if he gets in trouble doing this.

The child with strong Metal Element energy can intuitively grasp situations and quickly come to conclusions and form personal opinions. He is ready to learn, can evaluate quickly what is taught, and can turn the information into useful and applicable knowledge. He is the little professor in the group, who "gets to the point" meticulously and with analytical precision. In his actions, he can be very persistent with a sword-like approach that cuts right to the finish line. When a goal is within his developmental capacity, he has a notable self-discipline in carrying out the task. If new information is presented that changes some of the plans in process, he incorporates this knowledge and makes the best of the situation to complete the task.

Recognition and respect is important for a developing child with this nature. The child with a strong Metal Element influence openly shows his strengths and weaknesses and innocently expects respect for this. In this regard, he is tolerant toward the weaknesses of others and stands up for them if others do not. He knows right from wrong, what is fair and unfair, and what is honorable. This child often makes it his duty to see that everyone is treated fairly in a group.

He allows himself to be inspired by new ideas, once he has assessed their value for himself. When meeting new people, he has a knowing sense of who lives up to these values and stays away from the children who do not. Children with this quality feel themselves equal to their moral values and feel a positive self-worth as they recognize the importance of what they accomplish in the presence of these beliefs. When their opinion or assessment of a situation is called for, they are never at a loss for an answer, and give this in a diplomatic and tactful way when the Metal Element is in balance.

There is another sort of order that is significant to this child, namely that of rhythm and timing. The sense of timing in walking, speech, and dancing, of harmony and rhythmical movement, belongs to the strengths of strong Metal Element expressions. Even the timing of the changes of emotions and feelings that have to adapt to various situations in life find appropriate expression without being repressed or excessively vented when the Metal Element is in balance.

Nicky was five years old and entering his first year of kindergarten. He was excited for school to begin and had his mother read the list of what was needed for the first day so he could help her remember what he should bring. After one reading of the list, he kept a mental memory of what needed to be gathered and he counted the days with his mother until school began. He insisted on a plan of when they could shop or get his items organized and in order to bring to school. He laid everything out and put them in his new backpack in the order on the list. His mother commented on how organized he always was and how she needed to be punctual and stay with the plan she laid out with him when he was preparing for big events like this. On his first day of school he came home with a smiley sticky note and star for being organized and bringing everything to school that was needed. The teacher remarked on the take-home sheet that Nicky was orderly in his new desk and was the first to remember all the rules she had laid out for the class activities and behavior. He got an extra star for correctly answering all the questions about the classroom courtesies.

Imbalanced Expressions of the Metal Element

When the Metal Element is distressed and out of balance during development, one of the first places this becomes apparent is in physical symptoms. The organs that have the most contact with the environment will be affected, namely the skin and the mucous membranes. The Metal Element offers support for the development of all personal boundaries. The skin is the largest organ of the body and the primary receptor for the sensory system to develop self-awareness. The mucous membranes are the contact to the outside world as they interact with the atmosphere, climate, and environment we breathe in. The two combined are the physical medium that the Metal Element works through in the development of self-awareness.

The skin plays a substantially greater role in children than in adults. It is where all contact is initially made and the primary sensory system that develops recognition of objects in the environment and interprets the quality of touch the child receives. It is the organ that innately rejects unhealthy stimuli—allergies, poor nutrition, environmental stress—in a child's surroundings. This is expressed in skin eruptions, eczema, and infections or dryness of the air passages (mucous membranes). When symptoms like these are repeated from infancy to young childhood, it is a sign that the Metal Element is struggling to develop.

If, by the time a child reaches kindergarten, the Metal Element has developed in imbalanced ways, other physical symptoms such as diarrhea, constipation, nosebleeds, habitual coughing, or asthma may appear along with a variety of behavioral signs. This child may sigh frequently and often appear sad or dejected. He may be withdrawn or blocked when meeting new friends. When other children try to make contact, he may respond with bossy, advising behaviors.

Typically, children with strong Metal Element expressions strive for high ideals and values. Children with imbalances in this Element often have ideals that are beyond their developmental capacity. As a result, none of the work this child does meets his expectations of what he has idealized as the outcome. For this reason, he has great difficulty completing any task because he is not satisfied with himself.

This cycle develops into a lack of self-worth and low self-esteem. An inner uncertainty leaves him vulnerable and he compensates for this by accepting others' standards. Without his own internal structure, this child is defenseless against strange influences and does not have the ability to push them away. His sense of order can develop into compulsive structuring. This can be expressed by developing an excessive concept of cleanliness or an exaggerated love of order. Above all, there can be an intolerance of the slightest interruption to his sense of order from the outside. He has a strong requirement for quiet and often confuses inactivity and waiting with finding the solution to a particular situation.

Children with Metal Element imbalances often choose friendships that create a lot of suffering because others dominate or belittle him. His dependency on outside influences to define his inner self-structures makes it almost impossible to distance or free himself from these disagreeable friends. On the other hand, he doesn't let others get close who try or want to help him out of such relationships.

In a child with Metal Element imbalances, an exaggerated righteousness and love of order and truth can be so strongly developed that he constantly makes his knowledge known and appears to be a know-it-all. He can also be dogmatic, rebellious against adults, or the tattle-tale as he excessively attempts to keep order. With playmates, this child is uncompromising and rigid, and acts very harshly in his judgments. The sense of duty in a child with Metal Element imbalances can become obsessive as he wraps himself up in trivialities, constantly focusing on the faults in situations. With this can also come a communication style that is sarcastic, pernickety, and even has an appearance of arrogance.

The ability to learn quickly and apply experiential knowledge in children with strong Metal Element tendencies can be misused when out of balance. Because of their lack of feeling their own structure within, they can sometimes take advantage of other children, by scheming ways to take the best for themselves. They can develop selfish and unkind behavior toward other playmates.

When this child is part of a group and new adults approach, he might immediately go to them and draw near in unpleasant and intrusive ways. This can lead to inappropriate familiarity for the child with personal boundaries too undeveloped to know right from wrong contact. Such children are at higher risk of abuse. Among friends, he oversteps the natural bounds of distance and does not respect others' efforts to pull back. All in all, a child with Metal Element imbalances is typically perceived as unpleasant rather than as a child with marked behavior patterns asking for help.

With his light hair and pale skin, six-year-old Manuel seemed very delicate and ethereal. His shoulders were hunched forward, which often gave him a dejected appearance. His mother reported that he had a lot of infections as a baby and always had a stuffy nose.

Since Manuel was an only child, his mother received many invitations to be in playgroups, mother–child gymnastics, and similar types of activities. In all of these, Manuel was extremely restless, and afterwards he whimpered for hours, something his mother did not understand at all. Manuel showed no interest in making sand pies in the sandbox. On the contrary, he made it clear that he didn't like the damp and squishy sand at all. Further, Manuel liked neither snuggling nor smooching, which often made his mother feel rejected.

At the suggestion of the teacher, Manuel was sent to join the Spiel-Räume (Room to Play) group at the children's clinic in Germany. He was referred because he didn't like many of the kindergarten activities, such as finger painting or modeling with clay. When the children would make something, Manuel expected his artwork to be perfect, and he was dissatisfied with anything less. It became apparent that, for his age, Manuel had strongly defined concepts of value, such as good and bad or beautiful and ugly. A further peculiarity was that he could not bear to overstep whatever limits the teacher set or defined. This was expressed with anxious questioning, such as "Is that all right?" or "Can I do that?" or "Is that allowed?"

When other children played ball, he would join them enthusiastically in the beginning, but then run away a few minutes later and sit quietly in the corner looking at a book. He also displayed similar behavior in group games, particularly when they became highly active—he could not tolerate noise and activity around him for long.

The first time he came into the play therapy group, he seated himself somewhat anxiously along the wall beside the door and then slowly began to take part in activities. Then he ran right across the room, sat down, and said, "I am not getting any air!" After a moment, he shouted, "I feel dizzy!" Somewhat later, he lay down on the floor and said, "They're destroying me!" In a later conversation with the mother, she stated that she suffered from severe asthma, but Manuel did not.

Environmental Influences on the Development of the Metal Element

Like the Earth Element, the Metal Element belongs to the Front Family and is highly influenced by the environment. With touch being the primary and first sense of an infant having contact with the world, Metal Element capacities arise out of the developed sensitivity of the skin and the way it made contact with the world and gave a child his sense of self. The skin is the organ or perception that belongs to the Metal Element and is the container that creates the boundaries for protection and individuation that is slowly discovered as the child has contact with the world. The skin is the organ of perception for bonding with others, making contact with others, and creating separations and distinctions from others. The function of the skin in infancy is the metaphor for the ever-expanding capacities of the Metal Element that a child gradually develops into. Metal Element qualities allow the dual process of self-awareness that recognizes that there is no separation from all of humanity through the breath but that there is separation with everything by being in one's own skin. Self-awareness that has the capacity to hold both of these realities is more available to children if they are supported earlier in life with a respectful attunement from the environment that allows individual needs to be nurtured and cared for.

When an infant's needs are respected, protected, nurtured, and cared for, a child has the opportunity to develop capacities for the awareness of boundaries and respect on many levels. A child's environment needs to demonstrate healthy boundaries in physical contact and relating with others, objects, animals, and physical spaces. Order, organization, and awareness of time and schedules offer boundaries of daily living that also offer children a sense of self in time and space.

Exercises
IS THE CHILD READY FOR METAL
ELEMENT DEVELOPMENT?
Movement Exercises
1. Touching and Sensing
The child lies on his back with his eyes closed and his hands resting, palms down, on the floor next to his sides. With the tip of a finger, the trainer/parent/therapist touches various points on the child's forearms and the backs of his hands. The pressure should be brief and fairly light. With open eyes, the child indicates the places that were touched.

QUESTIONS FOR ASSESSMENT

1. Is the child able to do the exercise without assistance?

2. Can he indicate the correct points?

3. How big are any deviations? (A half-inch to an inch is OK.)

2. Can I Get Through There?
The trainer and a helper hold a rope parallel to the ground. The children stand about three yards away from the rope. Each child can give directions for how high the rope should be held for them

to walk underneath it without touching it, but also with the smallest possible gap under the rope.

QUESTIONS FOR ASSESSMENT

1. This exercise shows whether the child has a sense of his own size. Can he make it under the rope without touching it?

2. Is there very little or a lot of room between the child and the rope when he walks underneath it?

Those children who often bump their heads have not developed out of the *Keiraku* enough to fully enter the Metal Element developmental stages.

If you answered no to any of the questions from Movement Exercises 1 and 2, the following exercises can be done to help further the development of the *Keiraku* in a 5–7-year-old child.

Keiraku Development Exercises
1. The Sprinter

a. The child stretches her arms out in front of her, making loose fists with her hands but with the thumbs separate and pointing up to the ceiling. The fists are about level with the hips.

b. Now the knees move alternately towards the fists. The speed can be increased and the breathing can become faster, but the back should stay straight without bending over or backwards. The fists should also stay level with the hips without lowering them to meet the knees.

2. Step by Step

a. In a room that's as empty as possible, place a chair with its back to the participants in the middle of the room. Then lay a rope three yards away from the chair. Now one child goes up to the chair, and then back to the rope that will now become the starting point. As he does this, he counts the number of steps he takes between the chair and rope.

b. Then the child is blindfolded.

c. The child takes the same number of steps towards the chair, and then stops; he takes off the blindfold and sees how far he is from the chair. The teacher/trainer can move the rope and then the next child can try his skill.

3. How Big Am I?

a. The trainer/teacher/parent lays various flat materials (carpet remnants, blankets, sheets of newspaper, cardboard, rubber mats, pieces of fabric, cushions, or whatever is available) on the floor.

b. Each child chooses an item and sits or lies down on it, trying to make her body fit on to the shape as exactly as possible.

4. I Have a Sense of Myself

This exercise can be done one to one or with a group.

a. Two children form a pair and are given a beanbag.

b. Now one child is "treated"—the child can choose whether to sit or lie down. Then she is given a massage with the beanbag, which is rubbed over her back, legs, and arms. The other child should keep asking the child being treated if the pressure is comfortable.

c. Then change roles.

d. To finish, ask what the places that have been treated feel like. Are they warmer or colder? Do they feel larger or smaller?

5. Who Can Tell What the Treasure Is?

a. Set out a selection of materials beforehand (beanbags, ropes, cushions, chestnuts, small, firm objects such as a golf ball or a wooden foot massager, and so on). Spread out four blankets or tablecloths around the room, and hide the objects underneath them.

b. The children sit around one blanket and try to find out purely by feel what treasures are hidden under it. Then they go on to the next blanket and try to find out what treasures are hidden under that one, and so on, until they have done the round of all four blankets. When all the children have guessed the objects, the covers are removed and the treasures admired.

c. To finish, use the objects to build a path from one blanket to the next, and the children have to balance along it.

6. Game with Drinking Straws

a. You will need dishes, drinking straws, and seeds that are larger than the diameter of the straws (e.g. chickpeas, butter beans).

b. Form two groups. The groups sit at opposite sides of a table. In front of each group there are four dishes. In the left-hand dish there are ten seeds, and the others are empty. Now the seeds have to be transported from one dish to the next by suction, using the straws.

c. The first group to transport all ten seeds into the right-hand dish is the winner.

7. Elephant in the Carwash

The children stand in opposite lines, quite close together. They each take a turn at being the elephant. When the elephant runs through the carwash, he bumps against the sides with his shoulders. With the other children rotating like the brushes in the carwash, the elephant is able to pass through. Like this, it's possible to get the big elephant through the carwash. You need to be vigilant as to whether or not children are able to tolerate this degree of close contact and that they do not get too rough when passing through the carwash.

8. Your Double

a. Place a big sheet of wrapping paper on the floor. If none is available, you can stick sheets of newspaper together. The child lies down on the paper and the trainer draws the child's outline on it. Then the child can get up and admire her shape. A lot of children are surprised at their own size. The child can then paint her "double," cut it out, and hang it up at home.

b. These figures are especially fun to do if they are made for several members of the family and hung up next to each other. You can also cut clothes out of colored paper or newspaper, and stick them on.

Overview

Expressions of the Metal Element in children

	Balanced expressions	Imbalanced expressions
Behavioral expressions	*The little professor* Quick and eager learner, analytical and systematic thinking, precise, rational, self-disciplined, quick thinker, tactful, enjoys following rules, finishes tasks, organizer, persistent, clear values, strong sense of fairness and honor, tolerant of others' weaknesses, accepting	*The know-it-all* Obsession with order and organization, has to "know it all," bossy, very opinionated, unforgiving, perfectionistic, hypercritical, self-condemning and judgmental, hard on themselves, selfish, scheming, unkind, stands too close or takes toys away, difficulty completing tasks, appears sad and dejected, sighs frequently, intolerant of noise and too much activity, sarcastic, pernickety
Physical expressions	Clear and smooth skin, symmetrical movement patterns, good sense of timing, tidy, neat appearance	Blemishes, dry skin, tendency to catch colds, asthma, bronchial infections, dry nose, nosebleeds, chronic stuffy nose, constipation, diarrhea, cold hands and feet, skin rashes

Metal Element developmental characteristics and expressions	Ability to know self-boundaries; ability to sense and respect the boundaries of other children, adults, and the environment; acknowledging of others' differences and weaknesses; clear sense of honor; sense of self-worth, can form self-values; knows right from wrong, good from bad, fair from unfair; good self-awareness, natural sense of order, good sense of timing	Lack of awareness in physical boundaries of other children and adults; blocked ability to make contact with other children; superficial and calculating; low self-esteem; expectations of self-performance beyond development capacity; gets into friendships that belittle or dominate

All expressions listed in this chart will vary according to age and stage of development.

Questions for Observation
THE ENVIRONMENTAL SUPPORTS FOR METAL ELEMENT DEVELOPMENT

1. How does respect for the child's expression of emotions, desires, needs, and requests show up in his life?

2. What kind of boundaries does this child have in his life and how are these boundaries presented and maintained?

3. How much permission does this child have to "breathe" or express himself in his home, school, daycare, or friendships?

4. How is discipline implemented in this child's life?

金

5. How much loss has this child experienced in his life and how much room has he been given to express this loss in his developmental capacity?

6. How much room does this child have to say "no" or create personal boundaries in his life?

EXPRESSIONS OF THE METAL ELEMENT IN CHILDREN—KINDERGARTEN AND ELEMENTARY SCHOOL (5–7 YEARS OLD)

1. Does this child have any respiratory problems or catch colds easily?

2. Does this child experience any allergies (i.e. skin, diet, breathing)?

3. Does this child have any skin sensitivities (e.g. wool, detergents, elastic)?

4. Does this child have a sense of personal boundaries and the boundaries of others?

5. How important is it for this child to feel respected by others?

6. How does this child show respect in his environment and for others?

7. How easy is it for this child to establish and defend his own personal space and boundaries?

8. Does the child realize when he is too rough with objects in the room?

9. How does this child respond to rules or discipline?

10. How does this child respond to situations when he feels that he or another person is being treated unfairly or unjustly?

11. How does this child respond to environments that are disorderly or without clear boundaries and rules?

12. How often does this child tell others what is right and what is wrong?

13. How does this child respond to getting rid of toys and clothing that are too small or outgrown?

14. How much space does this child need from other children and adults?

15. Can this child judge distance between his body and objects?

16. How judgmental or critical is this child of others and his surroundings?

17. How aware of time is this child in his daily routine in life?

18. How important is it for this child to have his living or working environment neat, clean, tidy, and organized?

Developmental Requirements of the Early Expression of the Metal Element

1. Respect for individual needs, ideas, and boundaries.

2. Examples of order, organization, rules, and boundaries in life.

3. Examples of fair treatment and consistency in treatment with boundaries and rules.

4. Safe and warm contact with others, with clear physical boundaries.

5. Opportunities to assign value and meaning to objects and experiences in life.

6. Opportunities to let go of objects and situations in life when ready.

7. Discipline with consequences that allow a child to learn, as opposed to punishment.

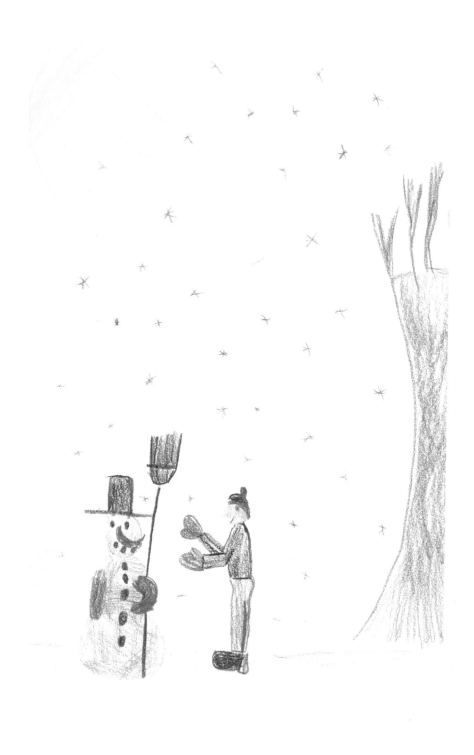

CHAPTER 8

The Water Element in Child Development

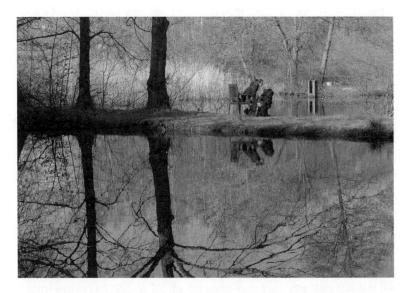

The Water Element gives us our will to live from deep within, and supplies us with the perseverance and steadfastness to ride the many turbulent waves and unpredictable circumstances in our lives. It is the spring and source that feeds all the other Elements with its capacity to flow and move regardless of what is in its path. It is a deep well that supplies the body, mind, and spirit with calmness and strength.

Water is soft and yielding, yet nothing can withstand its path over time. It offers us an ability to flow from one emotion to another and gives us tenacity to push through difficult times. The Water

Element is our energy source in life, constantly supplying what we need to maintain our course when we feel uncertain, undirected, and in between stages or transitions. It is a self-preserving power that guides us to rest and be still and silent so that the deep currents can be rejuvenated, rebuilt, and renewed. All direction, power, strength, and insight are born out of the deep calm Water Element and its ability to maintain the steady flow of the life energy for the body, mind, and spirit.

Adults
A Water Element Experience
The sound of the waves striking the shore can be felt throughout your entire body, and with every beat of your pulse you feel the tension dissolving. What a tremendous feeling, to listen to these endlessly returning waves! With a sigh of relief, you sense your relaxed body even more and allow the waves to flow over you. While you surrender to this feeling, a question comes into your mind: "What is in the ocean that makes it possible to relax so easily?" This question lingers for only a moment before the sound of the waves drives the thought away.

You lie back on the damp beach and feel the coolness of the water that washes over the beach. Sighing, your breath begins to deepen, flowing in and out without effort, merging rhythmically with the tide. All of your senses seem to follow the coming and going of every wave. You imagine that you are the ocean swaying between the sky, the ocean floor, and the beach. As you feel the weightless movement of the waves, you sense an unending force flowing from a deep source, and you realize this is the power of Water.

Your thoughts drift into wanting to feel more of the sensation of this invisible force and power. So you rise and enter the water, slowly moving through the waves, swimming away from the shore. The deeper you go, the more intense the movement becomes and the darker the water gets. You dive under, searching for the most powerful part of the movement and current so that your body can feel its strength. No matter how deep you plunge, the darkness extends still further into unknown depths, into a boundless space. You feel an eerie sensation as you realize you are surrounded by the cool, infinite darkness. You surface, check your distance from the shore, and relax on to your back as the water rocks and suspends you in a weightless peace. You savor the sensation your body feels as the constant movement of the water flows around and gives an impression of permeability and movement deep within.

You close your eyes and feel the entire ocean, from its surface to the dark depths below you. You feel the shore that meets the waves and acts as a support for the power of the water, and you experience the source that moves the ocean and tugs on the shore. Ocean and shore dance together between the pull of the moon and the spinning of the planet. The life that lives in them and on them are part of this powerful dance; everything is touched, swayed, rocked, and moved by this unseen force.

The penetrating cry of a gull reminds you that you are floating on the water. You open your eyes and slowly glide back to the shore to lie on the beach. You can still feel the rock of the waves in your body as you rest on the solid ground. You sit up, survey your surroundings, and sense the peaceful rhythm of the ocean within.

Expression of the Water Element

Adults with strong Water Element characteristics are those who have the capacity to endure experiences and tasks in life with a steadfast nature. They are like a great barge on the water, never faltering from their course as they travel from one side of the world to the other. As colleagues, they are those who calmly, humbly, steadily, and persistently perform their work. Their wardrobe would be simple, comfortable, and appropriate for their environment, classical in deep blue or black.

If balanced in their strong Water Element presence, their back would be strong and straight, and yet have a flexible, subtle appearance. They may even be involved in yoga, Tai Chi, martial arts, or other physical activities that call on deeper sources of strength and offer rejuvenating effects to the body, mind, and spirit. They walk at an unhurried pace, their gait appearing smooth and graceful. The movements in adults with strong Water Element expressions usually appear thoughtful and deliberate.

水

Other balanced Water Element characteristics appear in their mannerisms and way of being in a group. They often have a serious and straightforward reputation. Reserved and sharing only what is necessary, they usually do not volunteer personal information unless asked directly. On the other hand, they have a wonderful ability to listen. A shared secret is kept safe with one who has clear Water Element characteristics.

In a working environment or in circles of friends, this person is prized for her ability to listen to large and small problems and is called on often to do so. It is just this capacity to listen, without asking questions or giving advice, that encourages others to confide their deepest thoughts. A person with strong Water Element characteristics has the ability to wait patiently, enduring lengthy pauses in conversations, and, in that way, convey to the person having a conversation with her the sense of being taken as a whole person, without any value judgment, and of being "really heard" by her.

This ability to listen, combined with a corresponding reserve, nevertheless holds a danger that co-workers and friends may take this ability for granted. It is easy to forget that a strong Water Element individual is also a person with needs. It is then all the more astonishing to others when, in response to unfairness towards another—perhaps when a colleague is being run down, or someone else is being falsely blamed for something—an individual dominated by the Water Element speaks up powerfully and stands her ground for truth. This example of straightforwardness gives others courage to look inwards, even when the ensuing truth is unexpected or uncomfortable. Here the saying holds true: "Still waters run deep."

Imbalanced Water Element characteristics show up in adults in many opposites to the above descriptions. Often, individuals with significant weaknesses appear pale, look weak, and have constant back problems and poor posture. Their shoulders may be rounded and they are prone to be very sensitive to the cold. Individuals with this tendency typically have a shawl or sweater constantly in their possession to keep them warm.

水

Listening would not be their skill in life, appearing so withdrawn that they are inaccessible for others to talk to them. Physical impairment of the ears from strong constitutional deficiencies in the Water Element could exist. When spoken to, they may be impatient with the problems of others, showing signs of pessimism and sarcasm since they lack the energy to deal with their own problems. In a work environment, they would be those who get sick easily and, when an inconspicuous opportunity arises, complain about the energy drain others are creating in a company. Their inner monitor for balanced output of energy is often impaired and they will have a tendency to work beyond their physical capacity to experience a cycle of overwork and illness.

Correspondences and characteristics of the Water Element

Season	Winter
Climate	Cold
Tissue/body parts	Bones, teeth, bone marrow
Bodily fluids	Saliva
Orifices	Urethra, anus
Sensory organs	Ears
Sensory function	Hearing
Taste	Salty
External, physical form of expression	Hair of the head, teeth
Balanced behavioral expressions	Tenacious, persistent, constant, deep presence, ability to be silent and allow stillness, ability to rest, courage to allow new situations, seeks the unknown, adaptable, careful, modest, perceptive, reflective, sensible, objective, good listening skills, strong will

水

Behavioral expressions under stress	Anxiety, fearful of new situations, phobic, miserly, fear, panic, pessimistic, sarcastic, catatonic, withdrawn, demanding, blunt, penetrating, hermit, keeps to self, depressed
Balanced physical expressions	Steady, constant energy flow, good stamina, strong and straight spine, good fine motor skills
Imbalanced physical expressions	Poor fine motor skills, urinary infections, kidney or bladder stones, weak and stiff spine, loss of hair or premature graying, dark circles under eyes, tense, over-reactive, no stamina, infertility, painful menstruation, scoliosis, low back pain, chronic fatigue, tinnitis
Strength	Capacity to shiver (setting free from anxious energy and tension)
Verbal expression	Sighing, moaning, grumpy

Children

Expression of the Water Element

Calm and serious, a child with strong Water Element expressions is always busy with something. He pursues his interests steadily, and this shows in his stamina and steadfast manner when doing activities. His patient and enduring way of doing things gives others a secure feeling as if they are in a protected space.

Frequently, he removes himself from the group and sometimes wants to be alone, or simply to wait, but this behavior can be followed by spirited behavior that is appropriate to different situations. His sure demeanor and his courage to deal with disagreeable moments and their consequences shows that he has a sense of his own strength and can rely on it. A child with well-balanced Water Element characteristics is adaptable and able to submit when called on. But he also has a strong will that allows him to persevere and hold on to a desired goal.

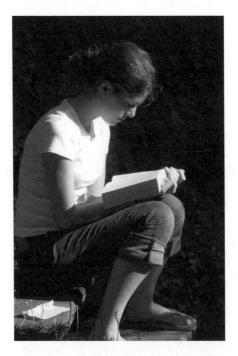

The child with strong Water Element tendencies doesn't need to brag about his knowledge and capacities. He often gets recognition and affirmation by unexpectedly astonishing and amazing others. There is a "secretly cunning little fellow" underneath the assured presence, and he knows how he affects others, just as he also knows his own weaknesses. Most often, however, he shows his serious, steady side.

The child with well-balanced Water Element development keeps secrets well, and others gladly place their trust in him. He radiates so much security and understanding for the needs of others that they often feel no need to compete with him. He doesn't emphasize his individuality and finds it disagreeable to be conspicuous.

Books and the cozy retreat that accompanies reading, or consistent puzzling with technical, fine motor activities, offers the Water Element an opportunity for internal concentration and are thus a source of inexhaustible energy. Children with these strong tendencies sleep well and can relax well. In bodily contact, it's easy for him to let go—he feels himself carried along with the attention.

水

A straight, upright posture is often a Water Element characteristic and an attentive liveliness during quiet activities. In sports, he belongs to the long-distance runners rather than the sprinters; he appears steadfast in any game and does not become exhausted easily.

The Water Element is recognizable very early in a will to survive—that is, in premature or severely disabled children. Often, against all statistics, these children will survive extreme birth defects, surgeries, and illnesses that other healthy children would not. They also exhibit a patience and undying will to learn skills that they were not born with the potential to develop.

One Water Element quality is primal fear, and children born with immediate physical and developmental challenges often face and experience this right from the start. The counter-attribute of primal fear in the Water Element is fundamental trust, a quality readily seen in the perseverance and steadfast nature of the survival will of children with disabilities.

Brad was a seven-year-old soccer player and one of the youngest players on his club soccer team of seven- to eight-year-olds. In spite of his smaller size and lesser experience compared with some of the other star players on his team, he was often the first child on the field for every game and the last off the field. He was known as the "Energizer Bunny," the player that kept playing steadily and never slowed or faltered in his energy level—like a battery that never runs down. He was not the fastest player on the field or the most accurate, but the coach could rely on him to stay in the game and run the ball up and down the field, passing and intercepting when needed. He was calm and steady, and normally didn't get emotionally ruffled when players from the other team pushed or jeered at him and his team mates. That is until one day when one of his best friends was tripped intentionally by a bigger player on the other team who stood over the boy and jeered at him when he didn't get up, holding his arm and crying in pain. Brad, knowing the seriousness of his best friend's pain, ran out on to the field and stood tall and wide in front of the bigger bully and, with a clear, loud, booming voice, told the bully to "Back off, and step away." So shocked were the coaches on both teams at Brad's powerful stance that both ran out on to the field as the bully cowardly backed off and away from his friend. His friend was taken to the hospital where he was found to have a broken arm; the team patted Brad on the back for standing up for his friend. Brad unassumingly let the team acknowledge him but quickly resumed his normal calm composure after the event as if nothing had happened.

Imbalanced Expressions of the Water Element

When the Water Element is out of balance, it shows itself in a lack of trust in one's own strength, one's own desires, or one's own reasons. Such a child goes the way of least resistance, placing herself in situations where she will not stand out, where she will not have to be accounted for, or will take up the least amount of space. Friends cannot rely on what she says because her exaggerated need for security leads her to change her mind frequently.

Like the winter months, where life appears to withdraw from the world, so can a child with Water Element imbalances. This can occur with varying degrees. A child may become introverted and move into self-isolation, retreating deeper inside herself. Unlike the healthy results of the restful winter months, however, where the earth renews its energy for spring, the retreat that comes with the Water Element imbalances is not a constructive quiet time from which something grows. Rather, a child with this behavior feels powerless and exhausted, and has little energy for activities that demand endurance. There can be a lack of spirit, feeble drive, extreme sensitivity, constant weariness, and a vulnerable delicacy that can isolate her from others.

She groans and whines a lot, anguishes over what is past, or holds fast to what is already settled. Once engaged in plans or arrangements, she has great difficulty accepting changes. Similarly, it is difficult for her to come to terms with changing facts if someone makes a mistake in a conversation and tries to correct themselves.

Lack of balance in the Water Element makes it difficult for a child to assert her own opinion or to show backbone in conflicting situations. Instead, she relies on tricky behavior or manipulation

水

to get what she wants. The German expression "mit alle Wassern gewaschen" ("washed with all waters") implies "knowing all the tricks." Devotion and closeness are usually superficial. Apart from the actions of withdrawal and self-pity, she gives few signs that could unlock deeper feelings. It is important to see that these behaviors arise from incapacity and not a conscious stubbornness, withdrawal, or decision to withhold devotion and closeness in her life. This falling into a kind of darkness or reactive space is usually related to an inability to find clarity in the depths of what is occurring.

The list of potential bodily symptoms in Water Element disturbances is long and includes any type of back problem— swayback or scoliosis being two very common forms. Slowed-down reactions, poor coordination in fine motor skills, bladder problems, cold feet, constant urinary pressure or nocturnal enuresis are the classic signs. Hearing problems can occur, along with disturbed equilibrium. The bodily appearance shows poor posture, sallow skin, and circles under the eyes. Such a child seems to be constantly cold. Other people want to take him in their arms, yet it is hard for him to relax with close body contact. Relaxation is essential, however, to develop an inner quiet as the source of new energy.

Tobias, five-and-a-half years old, came to the German Spiel-Räume (Room to Play) play therapy group for the first time accompanied by his six-year-old friend. He was sent to the play therapy group as a result of his fearful behavior in school which appeared to be associated with a hearing impairment he had since an earlier age. The other children, who had all been there before, were excited to be at the group and immediately came running into the room. Tobias clung anxiously to his mother's arm, cried, and didn't want to enter the room. With this, his mother came into the room and sat on the floor with Tobias. Tobias rolled himself up very small and covered his eyes and ears, without holding on to his mother. The other children had already returned to their different activities when he began to peep out repeatedly between his fingers.

Gradually, he became so interested in what the others were doing that he could not stay in his place, and slowly and carefully he approached the activity of the group. Little by little, the mother could then leave the room. Several children were pretending to be animals, and when Tobias was asked what kind of animal he would like to be, he answered, "A nobodyanimal— it's completely invisible and no one can see it, but it can be everywhere."

In the next two groups that he attended, it turned out that he could hear very well, and even had an over-sensitivity to noise levels. Also noteworthy was the persistence with which he completed things, which was accompanied by unusually good fine motor skills. He always had cold feet, and because of this needed extra thick socks, preferably two pairs on each foot. He was constantly going to the toilet, although only a few droplets came out. His posture had a marked swayback and an overall appearance of a stressed back. The visible tension increased when the other children expected an opinion from him during the group activities. New and unexpected things made him pull back and withdraw for periods of time.

Environmental Influences on the Development of the Water Element

Like the Fire Element, the Water Element differentiates out of the Back Family and the *Keiraku*. From infancy onwards, the Water Element needs a special kind of listening from the parents and caretakers that allows the innate nature of the child to rest, sleep, eat, and wake up according to her own rhythm and cycle as she acclimatizes to the world. Creating schedules that are consistent with the child's needs for rest, activity, food, play, and sleep supports a child to come into herself and find her natural flow and regulation of her life *Ki*. The Water Element is where the energetic resources and ancestral *Ki* are stored and released for the whole body to survive. It has a flow that can be steady and constant, and the quality of the flow of *Ki* is individual to each human being. Everyone needs to know when to rest, when to sit, when to be silent, and when to retreat into relaxation and quieter spaces. When infants and children are allowed to rest when needed and be still or quiet, a healthier expression of

水

the Water Element can develop with an intact self-awareness of what is needed to maintain balance and a steady flow of the life *Ki* to the body and activities. Rejuvenation and regeneration of the *Ki* is vital for human health, and it is the Water Element that regulates these needs for both activity and inactivity in life.

There is a container or ground needed for a healthy Water Element to develop, and that container needs quiet, safe spaces where an infant can rest without being startled out of her sleep. It is important for Water Element development that a child is able to rest without being on guard for unknown disturbances. Holding and contact, with support on the back of an infant, is also part of the healthy container needed as this creates a support for the needs of human beings to be held and have contact with others. Having basic human needs met, without alarm or deprivation, develops the initial stages of trust in a child. That trust is the foundation for confidence that the outer world can meet one's needs, which develops into inner confidence that one is acting appropriately for one's needs to be met.

Listening for the subtle needs of an infant and child is a form of support. When a child is listened to and allowed to express herself with impulsive excitement or retreat to quieter spaces and be alone, a child gets to know herself and can learn to monitor her energy levels. The more she gets to know herself, the more secure she feels about herself, and an internal strength develops that allows her to stand upright in the world with self-confidence. A strong sense of self-acceptance allows a child to rest deeply within herself, or move out forcefully in response to what is needed in the environment.

Exercises
IS THE CHILD READY FOR WATER ELEMENT DEVELOPMENT?

The main tasks of the *Keiraku* development that prepare the child for the Water Element are concerned with the development of the back of the body which gives the erect posture and initiation of movement. These specific *Keiraku* develop the sense of when the time is right to go forwards and when it's better to draw back, and how and where your own body is in space.

Movement Exercises
1. Walking Backwards
Cut a strip of carpet 6 inches wide and 3 yards long. Or you could draw a line on the floor.

"Try to walk backwards along this strip. But you can only put one foot down behind the other, not one next to the other."

QUESTIONS FOR ASSESSMENT

1. Can the child accomplish the task without looking behind?

2. Does he keep both feet on the strip?

3. Can he do this without making balancing movements (e.g. with his arms)?

4. Can he do this without making "rowing" movements (with his arms)?

5. Can he do this without needing help with movements of his tongue?

2. Sitting Stretch
The child sits on the floor with legs outstretched. He is instructed to touch his toes while keeping his legs stretched out.

QUESTIONS FOR ASSESSMENT

1. Can he touch his toes with his fingertips, and keep his legs stretched out?

2. Can he touch his toes without hunching his back over or pulling his shoulders to his ears?

If you answered no to any of the questions from Movement Exercises 1 and 2, the following exercises can be done to help further the development of the *Keiraku* in a five- to seven-year-old child.

Keiraku Development Exercises
1. It's Getting Icy
This exercise is better suited to a group.

水

    a.   "Move freely around the room. As soon as you hear the gong, you turn into a pillar of ice and stand there without moving. After a long or short interval you'll hear the gong once more, and you can move freely again."

    b.   Here the trainer can observe:

        1.   Can the child pause instantly?

        2.   Does she always assume an identical posture?

        3.   Does she copy the movements of the child nearest to her?

        4.   Does the child move without knowing?

        5.   Can she stay in this position, or does she wobble or even fall over?

Look for the ability of the children to do this fun game without any of the behaviors in the questions to observe the maturing of the *Keiraku*.

2. Secret Post
This exercise trains the fine motor skills that are attributed to the Water Element.

    a.   You will need an envelope that you have prepared in advance. Using a candle, carefully singe the envelope in one place.

    b.   The children sit in a circle, and each gets a wooden clothes pin.

    c.   "I've rescued this envelope from the fire and it's still quite hot! This means it can only be passed along with a clothes pin."

    d.   The envelope is passed from one clothes pin to the next with the children around the circle.

3. The Dancing Feet

    a.   This exercise can be done with one child or in a group.

水

b. The partners sit opposite each other with the soles of their feet touching, and "bicycle" together—sometimes forwards, sometimes backwards; sometimes slow, sometimes fast.

c. If this goes well, you can introduce the following variation. To the rhythm of a piece of music, one child leads the foot dance while another follows. It's important that the soles of the feet stay in contact. Then switch roles, and the other child takes the lead.

4. How Strong Am I?

Two children sit back to back and place their feet flat on the floor. Now each child tries to push or shove the other off their place.

5. Beware—Mice Can Hear in Their Sleep!

a. One child plays the mouse and sits on the floor with eyes closed. The other children are the cats and stand a little way from the mouse.

b. "You are the hungry cats and creep up to the mouse, one after the other. But beware! The mouse has good ears—as soon at it hears a sound, it squeaks!"

c. With eyes closed, the mouse points in the direction of any sound it hears. If it's pointed in the right direction, the cat has to go back to where it started. The cat that touches the mouse plays the mouse next time round.

6. The Magic Word

We have included this exercise with the Water Element because its main focus is on hearing and correct listening (although the other Elements also play a part in the wide range of movements in this exercise). This exercise can be done individually as well as in a group.

a. The children walk around the room and the trainer makes suggestions for movements to do. However, the children only carry out a movement if the magic words "Simon says" are said first: "Simon says, everyone walk backwards!" "Simon says, everyone roll around the room!"

    b. But if the trainer says "Everyone do a somersault!" then the children mustn't do the movement, since the magic words are missing.

7. The Flower Opens and Closes

    a. The children roll up into balls on the floor. "As soon as you hear the gong, the flower can open slowly and stretch towards the sun." The trainer/teacher/parent rings a gong and lets the children open slowly towards the sun.

    b. "There—and now it's evening again" (announced by the next stroke on the gong) "and the flower closes up again."

8. Which Creature Has a Home?

    a. Each child is given a blanket and asked to fold it up small enough to fit on their back (the children may need to help each other). The trainer says to the children, "What animal are you today? What would you like to be? Let yourself feel the legs, arms, and body of that animal and move on all fours around the room the way that animal wants to move and go."

    b. "Now the animal is getting tired and crawls back to its home. Find a spot and let your animal crawl back into its home, making yourself nice and small, where it is dark and comfortable."

    c. The trainer/teacher/parent rings a gong or bell after a few minutes and tells them to slowly come out again, stretching their heads and feelers out of their home, and move around the room once more.

9. Sensing Your Own Body

    a. The children lie flat on their backs on a blanket. "How are you lying on the floor? Which parts of you are touching the blanket and which are facing upwards? Now bring both feet slowly towards your bottom and pause for a moment—then you can slowly stretch your legs out again." Repeat two or three times.

水

b. "Now, really slowly, move your feet towards you and put them flat on the floor. Now lift your right leg up and put it down on top of the knee of the other leg. Can you feel your left knee pressing against your right calf? Now increase the pressure a bit, but only as much as is comfortable for you. Then you can ease off the pressure again. Now do the same with the other leg."

c. Next, the children have to clasp their knees with both arms and press them towards their tummies.

d. "See whether you can increase the pressure. How does it feel? And now lift up your head. Now you are a bundle tied up! Try rocking to the left and to the right—try out all the possibilities."

e. Then the children have to let go of their legs and put their feet on the ground again, and slowly let their legs slide back into extension.

f. "And now feel yourself lying on the blanket!"

g. The exercise can be extended by having the children lie on their sides and once more draw their legs up to their chests with their arms. At a stroke of the gong, still lying on their sides, they stretch out full length, stretch out their toes and fingers as far as they can, then roll up again into bundles, lying on their sides. Then they roll over on to their backs and wait for a few breaths, before doing the same exercise lying on their other side.

10. The Sleeping Princess/Prince

This exercise can also be done with one child as well as in a group. Depending on the number of children, split into pairs or groups of three or more children.

One child plays the part of the sleeping princess/prince and lies down on her or his back. The other children sit around the princess/prince. Then one child begins, and carefully lifts up the princess's/prince's hand or leg and puts it down again. Then the next child lifts a part of the body. The sleeping princess or prince remains quite

水

passive and can't be disturbed. *Important:* only let one child touch at a time.

11. Distance Throwing in Reverse

The children form pairs. One partner sits on the floor and the other stands behind him. The seated child picks up a beanbag with his feet and rolls on to his back, throwing the beanbag backwards (over their head) with his feet as he does so. The partner standing behind him tries to catch the beanbag. Do this five times, then change roles.

Overview

Expressions of the Water Element in children

	Balanced expressions	Imbalanced expressions
Behavioral expressions	*The clever one* Persistent, calm, steady, willful, good listener, courage to allow new things, ability to relax and rest, seeks information, curious	*The over-persistent one* Exaggerated need for security, demanding, skilled at finding the path of least resistance, manipulative, lack of will, no stamina to act, over-reactive, nervous, anxious, fearful, introverted, withdrawn
Physical expressions	Good stamina; straight, flexible, strong back; ability to rest and sleep well	Frequent urination, sense to urinate with no real need; scoliosis; easily fatigued, poor stamina; water retention; tense; over-reactive; circles under the eyes; poor coordination; neurological system diseases; back and bone problems; problems with the teeth

Water Element developmental characteristics and expressions	Balanced autonomic nervous system, self-sufficient, ability to observe and introspect, sociability, ability to allow situations in life to flow, good fine motor skills	Inability to relax in new environments, lack of will for discovery, very fearful to try new situations or activities or meet new individuals, introverted, lack of trust, unrealistic determination, refusal to give up when necessary

All expressions listed in this chart will vary according to age and stage of development.

Questions for Observation
THE ENVIRONMENTAL SUPPORTS FOR WATER ELEMENT DEVELOPMENT

1. How much time and space does this child have to rest and be still in life?

2. What is the noise level like in the home, school, daycare, and play environments of this child?

3. What is the energy level of this child like throughout the day? Is there a time when she appears tired and has time to rest and be still?

4. Does this child have any fears and, if so, how does she respond to them?

5. How does this child like to share information about herself, and when she does, how is it received?

EXPRESSIONS OF THE WATER ELEMENT IN CHILDREN—KINDERGARTEN AND ELEMENTARY SCHOOL (5–7 YEARS OLD)

1. Does this child need quiet time during the day or does she avoid quiet time?

水

2. Does this child have any urinary problems or bouts of bed-wetting?

3. Does this child walk in her sleep?

4. Can this child copy the movement from one side of the body to the other side of the body?

5. Does this child deliberately and tentatively walk more slowly on hilly surfaces?

6. If the child is pulled backwards unexpectedly while sitting, does she jump and have a strong startled reaction?

7. Does this child use more force or power than necessary when doing different activities (e.g. cutting with scissors, drawing, walking, running)?

8. Can this child wait her turn in a group situation?

9. Is this child fearful to try new things?

10. Does this child become so absorbed in what she is doing that she doesn't notice when the other children in her group have moved on to other activities?

11. Does this child like to play with toys that need fine motor skills such as small construction sets or small, fine art materials?

12. Does this child have any back or bone problems?

13. How courageous is this child?

14. Does this child have any fears or phobias that have existed for longer than six months?

15. Does this child have dark circles under her eyes?

16. Does this child have any chronic problems with her teeth?

17. What is this child's response if a conflict arises in a group with another child?

水

18. Is this child able to try again if she fails at doing something new?

19. Can this child listen while others are talking in a group?

20. Does this child show stamina to stay with an activity or assignment?

21. Does this child have a tendency to isolate herself?

22. Does this child like to receive massages with strong pressure?

23. Does this child push other children very hard, intentionally run into other children, or intentionally make strong contact with other children?

24. Is this child able to sit still for a period of time?

25. Does this child have any speech problems?

Developmental Requirements of the Early Expression of the Water Element

1. Listening out for the individual needs of the child and meeting those needs when able.

2. Consistent schedules that meet the needs of an infant or child.

3. Enough rest for rejuvenation and relaxation.

4. Relaxing activities that allow the depth of self to be felt—for example, reading, meditation, sitting or lying in a field or hammock, puzzles, having stories read out loud, taking baths, floating in water, watching the snow fall...

5. Being held and rocked.

6. Quiet environments and moments of silence.

7. Permission to express and discover impulsive energy and retreating energy.

水

PART III

The Five Elements in Practice

CHAPTER 9

Examples of Five Element Imbalances in Children in Everyday Life

In this chapter we look at some everyday behavioral, physical, and emotional examples of children in various situations in their lives. We hope to give you a variety of examples so that you can begin to recognize correspondences to the Five Element imbalances and how we approach them. Very often, circumstances and life changes are much more complex. Even in some of these examples, we have chosen not to become too analytical when explaining all of the involved ways in which the Elements are arising. Please do not let this deter you from trying to begin working with little incidents and the basic knowledge of the Five Elements. The more opportunities you take to play with and apply the Five Elements in daily situations, the easier it becomes to experience the natural and logical presence they offer and the simple ways they can support you and the children in your life.

Wood

Two-year-old Josephine stands before her toy chest and looks upward. She wants a book. Suddenly, she cries, "Mama—book!" She only needed to stretch herself a little bit more to reach the book herself.

From the Five Element perspective, we see that Josephine has a goal, but no plan for how she could achieve that goal on her own. She is still in the *Keiraku* stage of development and has not developed the capacity to plan her physical movements but she has learned to direct her mother to get the goal for her.

Neal and Paul are sitting in the block corner and getting blocks of different kinds. While Neal chooses interlocking blocks to build his city, Paul starts playing with blocks of all different shapes and sizes. Because of the instability of the different shapes and sizes of the regular blocks, and Paul's lack of foresight in stacking the blocks, his city keeps collapsing before he can finish his design. Paul then decides he wants to share the interlocking blocks with Neal, but there are not enough to build two projects. They argue with very clearly articulated statements and eventually start fighting. The block area is now deserted, and the unused blocks are scattered everywhere.

In the above example, Paul was missing the capacity to sort out the jumbled blocks and stacking them in such a way that they could support one another. Planning and strategy skills are Wood Element qualities that are not as developed in Paul as they are in Neal.

A mother enters a bank, holding her three-year-old son by the hand and carrying her two-year-old daughter. As she leans over to set her daughter down, the girl moves her feet as though she's already running. As soon as her feet touch the ground, she starts to run across to the other side of the room.

"Stay here!" says the mother, and quickly pulls on the running harness she had put on the toddler. With one yank, the little girl is prevented from running further and begins to cry and scream. The mother gives a disapproving comment about her nature to run and in a scolding tone says she must stay by her side. As the mother approaches her daughter and a slack in the tension of the harness is felt, the little girl tries to run in every direction, screams excitedly, and eventually throws herself on the floor, refusing to get up and go where the mother tells her.

The mother picks up the raging and flailing child, and carries her over to a chair. Again, the moment her feet touch the ground, she starts running off across the room in the same direction as the first time. Her mother catches her again, and once more there is screaming on both sides. This process repeats itself several times.

Here we have a good example of a situation that clearly expresses characteristics of the Wood Element, but the child is still in the *Keiraku* stage of development. Even though the Wood Element is not developed yet, the awareness of Wood can be used to support the mother and child in the struggle. The toddler is very distinctly expressing her need to move and satisfy her curiosity. She has devised a plan that she is unwilling to abandon. Her reactions to the hindering of this plan—her screams, flailing, and temper tantrum—are classical examples of the emotional expressions of the Wood Element. This shows very clearly the force with which movements for exploration need to express themselves, because the primary developmental needs of movement are the foundation for the Elements to develop.

The reaction of the mother to her daughter's early Wood-like characteristics is determined by her own Wood Element expressions. The mother's expression of anger and frustration, and her controlling attempts to restrain her daughter's behavior, make it easy to see that there is a struggle between the mother and her daughter's developmental *Keiraku* needs which are the precursor for the Wood Element expressions to develop. The stronger the mother's Wood Element expressions come forward in her attempts to control and force her child to be the way she envisions her child should be, the stronger the child reacts with her own need to move so that her energy can develop. The desire to grow and expand in a child can be wonderfully relentless.

As adults, we all have difficulty seeing our own reactions in many of the Five Elements, especially when faced with conflict with our own children. In a situation like this, the struggle between the mother and daughter will continue and turn into more complex control issues if the mother is not able to learn about the developmental needs of her daughter.

The Five Element approach would be to let the mother know about the developmental needs expressed in her daughter's behavior and then to help the mother find outlets for her daughter to express her *Keiraku* energy. The bank scene example could be shifted quite easily by the mother permitting her daughter to move in the original direction she intended, while at the same time encouraging other playful movements and activities to help direct her energy more clearly.

The mother could, for example, suggest that the daughter direct her running over to the chair, or she could pretend to race her to the teller windows. She might stimulate her daughter's curiosity: "See that chair over there? Do you think there is something under it?" Another possibility would be for the mother to carry a variety of small items that would provide the little girl with something to do when they were running their daily errands. For example, a colorful scarf to wrap around her daughter's head could give the mother enough time to discuss her business with the bank teller or grocery store clerk. The point of offering different ways for the daughter to express her exploring energy is to open up new possibilities of movement which will allow her to mature and develop this very important aspect in her life. This little girl is in a phase of life in which her *Keiraku* energy is demanding room to express itself, a challenging time for even the most patient parents!

Fire

Allison was a strawberry-blonde little girl with bright blue eyes. She was known for her laughter, giggles, and wonderful lighthearted way of being silly. All her classmates loved her and her teachers just loved her light nature. When she was eight years old, her family moved away from the town where she was born and she had to leave her best friend who she had grown up with since the age of two. She wrote to her friend all the time, sent little gifts, and missed her very much. She got lucky in her eleventh year when her father was transferred back to the same town where her best friend still lived. She got even luckier when her mother was able to get her into her best friend's fifth grade class in the middle of the school year.

But Allison soon became very disappointed. Her best friend had been established in her school already for six years and no longer shared the same interests as Allison. Allison's mother reported that Allison complained about her friend all the time and said she acted too grown-up and didn't want to play the way they used to play. She began making nasty remarks to her friend at school while acting as if they were jokes. When Allison's friend confronted her, she would laugh and say that she was too sensitive and that she was only joking. The girls had terrible fights and shed many tears.

The strong Fire Element characteristics can be seen in Allison's lighthearted nature as a child who is loved by everyone. Her attempts to continue her relationship from a distance for three years also shows advanced expressions for an eight-year-old who might feel the loss but not have the full ability to follow through with the continued contact. When Allison returned, the friendship had not changed for her and she wanted to have the same kind of contact she had before she left. The change in her best friend touched her heart deeply, and the free expression of the Fire Element began to show that it was disturbed through the inappropriate humor and lack of ability to face the truth when confronted with the situation.

The whole class is bursting with laughter but the teacher, Mr Smith, looks unnerved and disgruntled. Sarah, ten years old, is sitting at the front of the class sneering. She has succeeded once again: she has gotten the whole class to laugh with her quick humor. This is her specialty. At the break, her classmates all come and pat her on the back for creating such a great moment in the class. Sometimes, she even gets applause during class time. Sarah appears to enjoy the acknowledgment and attention she gets when this happens.

The above is a classic example of a child expressing a Fire Element quality. The "class clown" syndrome is common, and very often these children are well liked by all in their classroom. Whether or not this behavior is an imbalance is a good question. If this behavior gets in the way of her expressing other qualities, and creates disharmony with her teachers so that she gets reprimanded but still repeats the behavior, this would be disharmony. Or if the humor is presented at inappropriate times, then we would say that the class clown behavior is showing signs of a Fire Element imbalance.

Leigh was two-and-a-half years old when her six-year-old brother began the Five Element program. During the brother's therapy, he got in touch with a lot of Wood Element energy that was not expressed when his little sister was born, and for the first two weeks he was upset a lot. Very suddenly, he would burst into tears and cry and yell at Leigh, and say that he did not want to play with her and wished that she was not there.

Leigh was typically a very happy, laughing, and smiling little girl with bright eyes, and her sunny disposition seemed not to be touched at first. She would not react to what her brother was saying and would go off and play with another toy or play with her mother who was trying to keep the peace and give her son's energy room to move. But after two weeks of this rejecting behavior from her brother, she began to stutter. Whenever she wanted something, she would point to it and begin the word of a sentence and get stuck like a broken record. Or she would get stuck in the middle of the sentence and not be able to complete it.

The above is a good example of the early development of the Fire Element occurring with an imbalance in the face of a shock and heart-disturbing behavior with the rejection. Leigh is in the *Keiraku* stage of development, and clear speech is the eventual development of the Fire Element. Even though this sunshine child showed no immediate reaction on the outside to the sudden behavior of her brother, her heart was still shocked. She felt an emotion without the ability to recognize it yet because she was still in the *Keiraku* stage of development. She could not communicate what she was feeling because this understanding was not developed yet. The foundation energy for Fire Element development began to lose its natural movement, which revealed itself in the blocked speech. She was seen by a homeopathic doctor right away and within three or four weeks the stuttering left completely. Her parents also supported Leigh by creating other play environments with fun playmates, and began to help her find ways to communicate what she wanted. Her brother also moved through his angry Wood Element expressions and, when it was necessary, was taken to more private spaces in the house to express his feelings about his little sister without her being present.

Earth

A family moved to a new house within the city. Their two children, aged three and seven, had lived all their lives in the old house. The mother reported that both children had begun to exhibit a whole new array of behaviors since the move. Her three-year-old son suddenly wouldn't leave her side and wanted to be carried everywhere, ate only from the plates of his parents, or wanted to be fed. He needed support in every activity, even in doing things that he used to be able to do without help from his parents. Additionally, he wanted to chew gum all day long. The seven-year-old girl also had become very clingy, always wanted to sit on someone's lap, and would sleep only in her parents' bed. If it were up to her, she'd eat nothing but sweets. Although she was always very creative in drawing, now she just wanted to copy pictures. She had become very concerned about little things that were previously unimportant to her. She complained of muscle cramps and unspecific pains. She would go to outside activities only when her parents were with her and she leaned against them when standing close.

These examples of behavior are all expressions of the Earth Element struggling with the changes from the move. It is through this Element that children develop a sense of feeling sure about themselves, sheltered, and supported in their existence. For children, a home is a stable ground that offers a sense of security and gives room for these qualities and inner senses to develop. When the living environment or other consistent environments change drastically in children's lives, they lose a trusted ground that was supporting development of the Earth Element expressions. This is what has happened to these two children. The younger child is still in the *Keiraku* stage of development, but the Earth Element in the holding environment changed, and the early independence and ability to step away from the parents regressed with the changes. One could say both children are feeling as if the "rug has been pulled out from under them" and they are regressing to earlier expressions and showing the need for stability in the Earth Element environment. The older sibling who was in the Earth Element stage of development lost her ground and sense of earth, and, instead of being able to express the Earth Element herself, needed the parents to feel secure and grounded.

From the Five Element perspective, it is important for the parents to allow these regressing behaviors to be expressed and to give the support they need. This will create a sense of holding so that the children can begin to experience the security of their new environment. It will take some time before the same inner security returns and they move back into their independent nature in their new home.

Three first-graders walk home from school together. When they reach the house of the first child, two of the three children go inside for a moment, while the third one waits outside the door for them to continue on their way home. But the child that is supposed to return outside doesn't come out. Gradually, the third child waiting outside becomes uneasy. He doesn't know what's going on inside and he also knows that his mother is expecting him at home. So he waits there, in distress, with tears running down his cheeks, unable to do anything to change the situation.

The above child is showing a need for more development in the Earth Element. He hasn't developed a strong sense of center and self-perspective, which makes it difficult for him to process or digest information in difficult situations. Not feeling strong in his own point of view—his mother was waiting for him to come home, he probably wasn't allowed to walk alone, and the idling of the child inside might get him in trouble—makes it difficult to think through the situation fully to figure out what action he needs to take. Instead, he is in an indecisive position, torn by three different possibilities: whether to go inside and find out what his classmate is doing, to continue on his way alone without waiting, or to wait longer.

From the age of five, Maya was extremely interested in gardening. So much so that her parents roped off her own little section in the family garden so that she could take care of this all by herself. She would sit for hours alone in the garden and just be happy with the butterflies and playing with the soil. She was not interested in playing with other children, because no other child was interested in the same things. But this did not bother her and it went unnoticed; as long as she could play in her garden, she was happy. She grew plants all year round and her bedroom was full of planters. She also loved to help with cooking and to be in the kitchen with her mother.

At the age of nine, she got her own guinea pigs. The most important thing for her was that they had babies. Every year she took care of them, and made sure mommy and the babies were well cared for. She never needed reminding to handle all of their needs; she was very disciplined and acted like a little mother.

As she got older, she became very interested in horseback riding, and her neighbors made an agreement that, when she took care of their horses, she could ride for free and get lessons. This consumed her whole world. She cleaned the stalls, brushed the horses, took them to pasture to graze, brought them in from the fields every evening, made sure the water and hay were fresh, and even hand-spun the hay for the barrels. At the age of 14–15 her day looked like the following. Before school she would get up and take the horses out to pasture and do the chores needed for them for the day. When she got home from school, she would quickly finish her homework and go again to take care of the horses and then go horseback riding. She had no contact with other teenagers because she was busy taking care of the horses.

The above is a very good example of how an Element can consume a child's world and dominate her expressions, and, at the same time, go unnoticed because the behaviors do not cause any problems for other children or adults around them. This little girl showed extremely strong Earth Element characteristics as a theme for most of her life. She loved to play alone, was very content doing so, and loved to garden, cook, and do caretaking jobs. But this Element expressed itself so strongly that there wasn't room for making contact with other children and learning other very valuable stages of development that come from relating and communicating with others.

Metal

Alison and Hailey were best friends from the age of two. They went to the same preschool and kindergarten and were in many ways like very close sisters. Despite attending different elementary schools, the friendship didn't falter and their mothers kept a weekly play schedule. This continued happily until the summer when they were seven, when something happened that was then compounded by unhappy circumstances.

Hailey was playing in the backyard with Alison and her dog. Hailey began to play as if she was "hunting" Alison's dog as she chased him on a tricycle through the yard. Alison got angry. She asked Hailey to stop, but Hailey went on doing it and laughed, because she found it so funny. When the babysitter intervened, Hailey claimed that she wasn't chasing the dog. This made Alison so furious that she burst into tears and screamed that Hailey wasn't her friend anymore and she never, ever wanted to play with her again. In spite of Hailey's apology, Alison refused to have anything more to do with her. Over the next couple of weeks, Alison constantly talked about the incident and adamantly refused to play with her friend. Then she began to paint pictures for Hailey, and wrote to her that she missed her. In tears, she explained to her mother that she didn't know if she could still trust her friend. After a while, Alison decided to play with her friend again.

When children reach a radical decision and set limits, we recommend that the whole environment of the child be observed. The above story has a background that was significant to Alison's family situation. Alison had two dogs, one of which was a Great Pyrenees dog that the family had raised for about two years and she loved very much. As the dog grew older and bigger, he became allergic to the tropical environment where the family lived. The family decided it was unfair for the dog to live in their small living space and tropical conditions, and had found a new home on a farm for the dog in a colder northern state. It was planned that he would leave the family in four weeks. It was during this time that the incident with Hailey happened.

Alison was confronted with two situations at once in her life that called on Metal Element energy. First, she was dealing with having to let go of a dog she loved very much, and, second, she felt she had to set some boundaries for her dog as Hailey was chasing him on the tricycle. For a seven-year-old girl, dealing with loss and letting go can be a very confusing energy, since she has not yet developed the capacity to comprehend fully the particular feelings that arise when parting from a friend or loved one. This energy was very present and looking for a way to express itself. The occurrence with Hailey gave her the opportunity to find a way of expressing the Metal Element energy—specifically, setting boundaries and letting go. The incident was tangible, in contrast to the confusing energy related to the upcoming departure of her dog.

Learning how to be with loss and setting limits and boundaries takes time and room to develop. To set limits, children need respect, time, and space. When the environment offers this, it gives them room to develop the skills to work with these difficult situations in life. As an adult in a child's life dealing with these issues, it is important to listen to their requests, offer them help, and guide them. Supporting their decisions honestly with warmth and compassion while allowing them to experiment with their limits will give them room—as in this case—to find the expression of forgiveness, another Metal Element quality.

Two mothers are talking outside the kindergarten room. One enthusiastically tells the other that she has just got two tickets to a Bob Dylan concert. Since this took some doing, both are rather excited.

Suddenly, a third mother joins in uninvited and remarks in a derogatory tone, "Bob Dylan? Who still goes to see Bob Dylan?"

This adult woman shows us an example of someone who has not developed a very clear sense of the Metal Element. This incident shows she lacks a sense of respect and boundaries for others.

Elaina was six-and-a-half years old and had two friends in the house playing with her while her babysitter was cooking and her mother was at work. A mother of one of her kindergarten classmates rang the doorbell and Elaina opened the door. The mother said, "I am leaving Katrina here while I go to my doctor's appointment." Elaina said, "No. There are already two friends here and it is enough. She can come another day." And she closed the door. Katrina's mother was very angry and went immediately to call Elaina's mother and tell her how rudely she had been treated.

The above example illustrates how a very clear expression of the Metal Element can show up in a six-year-old. Elaina was aware of her boundaries and felt that two children to play with were enough for her in her environment. She expressed this the only way she knew how for a six-year-old. This is also a good example of how adults may have inappropriate expectations about children's behaviors and how they express their emotions and boundaries. Katrina's mother did not recognize or respect Elaina's boundaries. By not asking before if it was alright to leave her child, she was also showing a lack of respect.

Water

Jeremiah has been attending first grade for eight weeks now, and is feeling the effects that this great change has had in his daily routine in life. His playtime in the afternoon has become shorter since his homework has increased. This afternoon, he has been sitting at the table for an hour and a half, writing his homework. But this takes a lot of strong concentration and effort because he writes each stroke of each letter very slowly as if painting a masterpiece. His back has become more bent during this time, and now he hunches over the table, appearing very withdrawn and weighed down by the homework. His mother notices his posture and demeanor and sits quietly beside him putting her hand on his lower back. Jeremiah straightens himself noticeably and suddenly finds the energy to write the last letters neatly in his notebook.

In the above example, the supporting hand of Jeremiah's mother on his lower back stimulated his Water Element quality, which gave him the strength to straighten his back and the stamina to finish the work. Since the Water Element energy governs fine motor skills, his handwriting comes to him more easily and accurately.

Melvin is three years old and has come with his mother to an appointment for her to receive a Shiatsu massage. Melvin brought toys into the treatment room and the therapist also had some children's toys that she took out for him to play with. For over an hour he sat beside the futon and played with his toys without one request. One particular toy that he played with was a bag that had many objects in it that stimulate the sensory system of children. Instead, he sat patiently and persistently for over half of the session, and very carefully, with a controlled index finger and thumb, delicately picked at the drawstring rope so that he could pull it out of the bag. He didn't look at the objects inside of the bag once before putting it down.

Next, he went to a small wooden box in the corner that was full of different-sized canisters that made all kinds of wonderful noises. He opened the latch to the chest, took one canister out and then put it back in the box, and carefully closed it by reattaching the latch. Then he was only interested in the latch, which again, carefully with fine little fingers, he closed and opened, closed and opened, closed and opened...for the rest of the session.

In the treatment, the therapist tried to make contact with him and he was very reserved. He only gave a shy smile once. The mother told the therapist that he was extremely afraid of adults he didn't know and until just a few months ago would immediately jump into her arms when someone came near. But he had gotten a little better with adults, although the fear remained with other children.

When he was born, his infancy was very easy for the mother. He was quiet, he played by himself, and when he wanted something would squawk only once or twice and then stop. He was a second child, and his mother was concerned that his needs were not being met.

Here is another child whose way of being in their early years is so easy that he is usually overlooked and not seen as having any imbalances at all. The warning signs here are his fears and his incredible patience at such a young age. His attraction to and skill at fine motor activities is very unusual. It is also important to note that he isn't interested in more movement and different objects in the room that would stimulate other sensory and motor abilities. He joined a Five Element play group, and his mother was amazed after two months at the change in his behavior and the missing part of the easy child she had before!

An 11-year-old boy went to a special children's doctor wanting to have his ADHD treated with alternative medicine. He was taking the prescription drug Ritalin, but had forgotten to take his medicine the morning before the session. He reported that when he did not take the medicine, it was very difficult to concentrate and sit still. He was extremely intelligent and reflective. He suffered from migraines and noticed that they came before a thunderstorm. When he got these headaches, his face became very pale, his head got very hot, and he had to stay in a dark, quiet room because he was so sensitive to light and sound. He said that he loved to go swimming, but every time he did he would get the same nightmares right afterwards. He always dreamed that he was drowning or that there was a spiral that was transporting him into the darkness.

His mother reported that when he was born, they had a very difficult birth. He was stuck for hours in the birth canal and the midwives were pressing on her stomach to help get him out. They were both in a life-threatening situation. Also, when he was four months old, he nearly died in a sudden death syndrome episode. She was in the kitchen cooking, and got a feeling that she needed to check on him upstairs where he was sleeping. When she got to the crib, he was lifeless and not breathing. She resuscitated him and he came back.

It is important to note that ADHD and migraines have many variations of elemental imbalances and Water is only one of the numerous possibilities of combinations that exist. For the above boy, ADHD arises out of a need to move and to feel that he is in his body. Water Element imbalances often include imbalances in the proprioceptive system, which has to do with the body sensing exactly where the joints are and the amount of pressure, tension, and movement that is needed in daily activities such as sitting down in a chair. His sensory system in this area was imbalanced, and his body had the need for constant movement to sense where he was.

This example is also very interesting because here we can see how early impressions and disturbances to energetic development may have occurred at the moment of birth. His dreams and brush with death twice in his life are noteworthy as well.

The Pinocchio Effect: Combinations of Five Element Expressions

The Five Elements will automatically adjust and express themselves however they can in an attempt to find stimulation for growth wherever the environment has an opening for the expression. Like a puppet, when you pull on one string to raise a leg, the rest of the body will shift and adjust to create some kind of balance to stand upright in the space around it. Children will take on regressed, precocious, over- or under-active behaviors of the Elements when needing stimulation for growth. As an adult working with children, it is always recommended to observe one's own Five Element expressions and to give room for the Five Elements to be expressed in the children around you.

Earth and Metal

A group of children are sitting peacefully snuggled in a corner with a teacher looking at a picture book. Everyone has a good view of the illustrations in the story. A young boy comes to join the circle but doesn't choose a suitable place as he tries to sit on the teacher's lap. After an interruption to the story and an argument with the other children, he is allowed to do this. During this new settling, however, two girls on the group stand up and go away, because they don't like the noise. The teacher continues with the story and the boy on her lap doesn't pay attention to the pictures or the story. It is clear that he only wanted the closeness and feeling of being held by the teacher.

The above boy reveals a need for more development in the Earth Element capacities with his need for holding and is able to get his needs met by playing on a Metal Element weakness in the teacher. This Metal Element weakness appears in the teacher's inability to create clear boundaries for the boy and boundaries that support the other children in the group. Other choices for Earth Element support could be offered to the child without disrupting the other children, like giving the child a beanbag cushion to sit on.

A first-grade class had free time and the children could do what they wanted for an hour. A group of children decided to play with a craft game and went to the middle of the room to get the supplies. Each took a reusable cork board that they used to create pictures with pieces of brightly colored wood in geometrical shapes. They would nail the pieces of wood on to the cork board with a hammer and special small nails, and, when finished, return all the pieces back to the center. Stephie took almost all of the nails from the art box and pushed them right away into her board. The other children tried to take one nail for each piece of wood to complete their project. Eventually, no more nails were available for the other children and Stephie had a lot left that she refused to share. The children started to argue with Stephie and all the children got in trouble.

The above is an example of how conflicts can arise when adults expect something from children that they are not ready to handle yet. The first grade teacher did not take care to first make the rules for playing with the art supplies and then she didn't make sure that every child got their portion of what they needed. In this situation, the lack of structure is a missing Metal quality along with the inappropriate disciplining, and the lack of caretaking or showing the children how to share in this game is a missing Earth Element quality. Also, Stephie herself is showing a need for more support in learning how to express the Earth Element, as this is where the natural tendency to care for others and sharing arises.

Metal and Wood

In a downtown café, where customers can listen to music and browse through books, two six-year-old girls, Andrea and Yasmin, stand painting on a huge sheet of paper. Both of them are deeply involved in this activity.

A third girl pushes her way between the two, makes room for herself at the paper, and begins painting over the drawings of the other girls. Andrea, on the left, stiffens, pulling her arms in close to the sides of her body, and does not resist being pushed out of the girl's way. With closely pressed lips and wrinkled brows, she watches what is happening to her painting. To the right of the "pushy painter," Yasmin stands, snorting and looking as though she's ready to boil over. As she stamps her foot, one can almost see clouds of steam above her head. All at once, she turns around and calls in a loud voice that carries throughout the café, "Daddy! Come here! That girl is painting all over my paper!"

In the above situation, Andrea shows a lack of Metal Element energy development. She isn't able to define her boundaries. When someone, without warning, forcefully pushes in on her space, she retreats into herself and gives up her place. The girl who pushed in between the two is also closely linked to this Metal Element theme. Without any thought of others, she oversteps the boundaries of both of the other girls and has no respect for their work already completed.

Yasmin has developed more of the Metal Element attributes, and this can be seen in her ability to recognize that her boundaries have not been respected. But her action comes out of Wood Element energy. The Wood Element expression brings her to boiling point, but then the "little general" prefers to call in her troops for defense. She herself would rather do the planning and supervision, and let her father take care of her boundaries.

Water and Fire

Eleven-year-old Eric came for his first appointment to a Five Element play therapy group on a warm autumn day. He was wearing gloves and a thick woolen cap that covered his ears. He had a very fair complexion and was very slim and tall for his age. He was Russian-born but spoke German impeccably, with no trace of an accent. He and his mother entered the therapist's room and his mother very energetically and enthusiastically took a seat while he stood some distance away from her.

Eric didn't even notice or look at the fun objects to play with in the room, even though there was a trampoline and other things that were normal for a boy his age to want to play with. His mother began the conversation by saying that Eric's school teacher had sent him to the Five Element group because she wanted him to learn how to act like a child. He was interested in only reading, math, and writing, and had no interest in movement or sports. When he did do sports, he got tired very easily.

The therapist asked him what he liked to do most. He told her that he most enjoyed having peace and quiet and being left alone.

The mother began to talk again and he interrupted her with "Excuse me, please, could you tell me exactly what I have to do in this group?" The therapist explained and his mother began again to try to talk. Eric again interrupted and said, "Excuse me, please, could you tell me the exact time the group begins and ends, and when I have to come?"

The therapist explained that she was very sorry but she didn't know which group she had room in, so she wouldn't have that information until next week.

Eric replied, "But I have to know exactly if I have to come next week, or in two or three weeks." This time the mother interrupted with an exasperated sigh and said, "Ahh, he needs to know everything exactly, and it must be done exactly as we spoke of before. He has a twin brother who is completely the opposite, like fire and water!"

It took a lot of talking with the therapist before Eric agreed to come to the first session just to see if he liked it enough to continue.

Eric's Water Element imbalances are expressed in his appearance and daily behavior. It is a warm day and he is dressed in heavy winter clothes; he is pale and thin, does not like activity, prefers to be alone like a hermit, gets tired easily with physical exertion, and is obsessive about having to know exact details for plans and gets upset if what has been promised is not stuck to.

His Fire Element qualities are the second level of expressions that reveal themselves as he speaks very politely and with precision, as if he were a well-groomed, socially practiced gentleman. This teacher's wish for him to learn to act like a child also suggests the playful, fun-loving vitality one normally sees in varying degrees in an 11-year-old boy is not being expressed in the Fire Element.

CHAPTER 10

Guidelines for Working with the Five Elements and Children

As shown in the examples in Chapter 9 of different children and their expressions of the Five Elements, children have come to us for physical, behavioral, sensory, and emotional reasons. Our work with children and the Five Elements for more than 20 years has evolved into many different settings where the range of our access to working with children has expanded from the original Spiel-Räume group play therapy in Germany to the classroom, parent or mentor education, and individual work with therapists including physical therapists, occupational therapists, psychotherapists, and counselors. We have been able to work with children in the natural flow of the learning and growth of the Five Elements as well as therapeutically with those who are struggling. This chapter will outline the focus and foundation that we still consider when working with children and the Five Elements, and offer an example of how to create exercises for children in different settings.

The primary principle that the Five Element work has offered us is the ability to see children in all of their states in life as in terms of temporary stages, either expanding naturally and without issues or attempting to grow as they seek the right kind of stimulation to help them access new behaviors to mature in the world. So our work with children begins with the way we view these children and their difficulties, struggles, or developmental leaps. We begin by seeing them exactly as they are, expressing what they are capable of at this time, and, underneath it all, looking for new opportunities to learn and grow. This perspective lays the foundation for every other aspect of working with children in a Five Element focus. There are two key features to consider when thinking about offering children ways to grow with the Five Elements. These involve the concept that growth happens inwardly and outwardly through stimulation and the environment.

- *Stimulation:* Adverse or troublesome behaviors and physical symptoms are viewed as repeating, stuck patterns in the Five Element expressions that know no other route for movement other than what has been learned. Most often, they are looking for stimulation to learn another way to move something that wants to expand inside. Children can only express confusion and expanding energy in the ways they have learned so far or the ways that the environment has offered them. To have access to new and more appropriate ways of expressing what is trying to grow, children need different choices, examples, and exercises to stimulate the Five Elements so that they can continue to develop new behaviors with more variations and possibilities. Something new must be offered in the environment for children to grow.

- *The environment:* Stimulation from the environment comes in many different forms—air, food, physical surroundings, schools, friends, family, mentors, teachers, and therapists. Everything children have contact with contributes to their total environment, from the *in utero* experience to the moment they are born and as they continue to develop in the world.

The box below summarizes what we consider to be the foundation of the Five Element focus needed for adults to be able to support child development from this perspective.

The Foundation of the Five Element Focus

To work with the Five Elements with children we must:

- see and accept children exactly where they are in this moment developmentally

- recognize that all physical, mental, sensory, and emotional behavior is an expression of the Five Elements in life and that this energy structure is inseparable from the process of development

- recognize that children are hungry to grow, expand, and learn, and that it is the function of the Five Elements to support and fuel this process of outward expansion and search for new expressions

- understand that everything in a child's environment—the air that they breathe, the food that they eat, the physical surroundings, and the people and objects that they have contact with—stimulates and affects the development of the Five Elements

- understand that children "act out" and develop anti-social behavior because the Five Elements have not learned another way to express the energy that is trying to move inside them; they are in a stuck pattern, trying to move an innate cycle that simply needs to expand and learn new patterns

- learn that balanced growth is possible when all five of the Elements have room to express themselves.

Entering the Five Element Focus with Children

If we can see children exactly where they are developmentally and boldly look at their behaviors in this way, it opens our view and removes our expectation of them to be something that they are not at this time. Our view creates a safe space and holding environment that we build by accepting every action as an attempt to grow. Here we have taken the first step to being a supportive part of the environment that is offering new stimulation for children to change and grow.

Working with children and the Five Elements quickly reminds us that the Five Elements are not something that is outside of us or only in the children we are focusing on. If we are part of the environment of the Five Elements, they are also in us and we are expressing our evolution of the Five Elements daily. We need to reflect on the Five Elements within us and the ways we express them as we work with children.

> All Five Element work with children begins with observing the self as part of the child's environment.

This concept became very clear as we worked with children and their Five Elements in different settings. As we focused on the children and their expressions, and as we played in exercises that stimulated the Five Elements, so too were we moved by this innate flow of energy. As we were moved, we could see the places where the Elements within us were also stuck in our own bodies and behaviors. As we continued to reflect and use our life experiences to broaden our own ability to respond in the Elements, so too did the Elements stimulate our inner network and expand our personal expressions beyond what we were capable of before. This naturally increased our ability to work with the children, who in return expanded and grew to find new abilities, expressions, and behaviors.

> The Five Elements are a *common ground* that we step into when working with children. Out of this arises a deep respect for all human beings, regardless of culture, race, or country of origin.

The Five Elements are a common ground that we must step into as we begin working with children from this perspective. It is a process of self-growth and self-evaluation that flows as easily as breathing in and out. It is a meeting ground where adult and child dance together, allowing the innate structure of the Five Elements to guide and move the process. Out of this common ground arises a respect and sense of connection to all human beings, regardless of culture or country. As we played in this common ground, we began to see that the Five Elements were much more than a therapeutic view; we experienced them to be universal and a root to humanity that represents an Archetypal Common Language that can be understood independent of a verbal language or culture.

> The Five Elements and their corresponding characteristics of behavior gave us a foundation of what we call an *Archetypal Common Language* that is independent of verbal language or culture. Here we found a way to understand how children express themselves and respond to their world around them.

As we worked together with children, this Archetypal Common Language helped us to understand their primal form of expressions and we could now decipher the ways in which they communicated their experiences and reactions to others. Their behaviors not only corresponded to the characteristics of the Five Elements but they also followed the natural cyclical pattern of the Five Elements. They would move through an exercise following the same flow and direction of the Five Elements. We call this natural-occurring pattern the Fundamental Rhythm of Life, and this innate rhythm and the characteristics that define its five aspects, or Five Elements, is the Archetypal Common Language.

> The behaviors of children followed a natural sequence that corresponded with the cycle of the Five Elements. This natural flow became what we call the *Fundamental Rhythm of Life*. It is the natural order in which we process our perceptions of the world and respond to our reality.

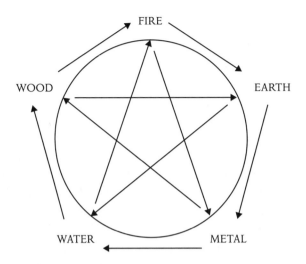

The cycle of the Five Elements, the fundamental
rhythm of an archetypal language

It is through sensing, observing, and playing in this fundamental rhythm of the Five Elements that we were able to reach a level of communication and connection with children that went beyond anything we experienced before. In the field of the Five Elements, we only needed to follow and offer exercises, games, movements, experiences, and sounds that followed the natural direction of the flow. The children's innate structure of the Five Elements responded to the stimulus offered, and they were drawn naturally to play in the Elements that most needed the energy and experiences to grow and learn new patterns of behavior, movement, and expression. As the children's energy in the Five Elements was stimulated and they played with simple games that inspired expressions and movements in their Five Elements, teachers, parents, and caregivers reported that anti-social and under-developed behaviors were shifting. Somehow the children had more abilities and capacities to respond to their home, learning, and social environments.

> When children are offered games and exercises that follow the natural order of the Five Elements, or the Fundamental Rhythm of Life, their innate structure is drawn to what is needed to grow and learn new patterns of behavior.

Play: The Fundamental Tool

The fundamental tool when working with the Five Elements and children is play itself. This is the gift and joy we have discovered with working with the Five Elements. Children are naturally drawn to the areas that need to be stimulated and they grow in ways that their inner network directs them. This happens repeatedly through the medium of play. Because energetic development is linked to the beginning stages of sensory and motor development, simple and playful elementary exercises can be used to stimulate the Five Elements. Play was a foundation of our work with the Five Elements.

In the Spiel-Räume (Room to Play) therapy center in Germany, children looked forward to coming to the classes; they were eager to do things that came naturally to them. The foundation of the Common Archetypal Language made it possible to decipher their reality and offer them exercises that were stimulating enough to move what was asking for growth inside. The more we offered them playful games, exercises, and activities that stimulated expressions in the Five Elements in the natural order of the Elements, the more they developed new abilities to respond to their surroundings outside the play therapy room.

> Play is one of the primary tools used in working with the Five Elements and children. It is the most natural medium for children to grow and learn.

When we talk about "play" in our work with children, we mean that the exercises and activities have an element of fun and room for the children's own creativity. Children learn and grow through playing. When they are given room to creatively add to play activities it supports the individual nature of what is trying to move and grow in a child. Games that involve movement of gross and fine motor skills, stimulation of the sensory systems, directing, planning, communicating, sharing, defining boundaries, and relaxation are primary themes when planning Five Element work with children.

The following examples offer simple illustrations of one type of exercise that we used in the Spiel-Räume (Room to Play) program for each of the Five Elements.

Examples of Games
Wood

The children use very big, geometric foam shapes to build a wall and put pillows behind it so that they can run through the wall and fall into the pillows.

This is a Wood Element game in several ways. First, we introduce the idea of building a wall to run through and ask the children to decide how to do this. Their own vision, decision-making process, and overall planning ability are stimulated with the creation of the game. The children have to have a vision to create the game. They make the plan of how to do this game. Then the children and teacher think about what they need to make the plan happen. They gather all of the large geometric shapes and pillows, and begin to build their own wall. This requires a lot of large motor skills and eye–hand coordination. They must build the wall so that it does not fall down. It takes a lot of strength and planning to make the wall tall enough so that they can run through it. When they are allowed to run through the wall, they get to experience how powerful they are that they can destroy this wall, and that they have the ability to build something again and again. If they don't use enough contraction in the muscles of their body when they run through the wall, the wall doesn't fall down. They really need to use enough strength. If they decide to run into the wall from a distance, they have to be careful with their direction so that they go through the wall and don't miss it completely!

Fire

This is a group game. All children wear loose socks and are instructed to crawl on their hands and knees through the room. Every child tries to catch as many socks as possible and keep them tucked in their waistband. After some time, the game stops and the socks are counted. Who has the most?

This is an example of the light, fun, and playful nature of Fire. Fire exercises have an element of speed for the participants to react with, and offer interaction with partners, contact and connection, a level of competition without any losers, and a lot of laughter.

Earth

Two partners stand on a piece of newspaper. Both stand on one leg and cross their arms with their hands on their elbows. Making contact only at the elbows, each child tries to push the other child off the newspaper page.

The Earth Element has to do with balance and being able to stand in one's place in the presence of others. This is a fun, physical activity which strengthens the core and encourages children to stand their ground in a playful way.

Metal

Draw a line on the floor. Form two groups of three or four children. All are on their fours in a crawling position. Each group has a balloon. Now they try to transport their balloon to the other side of the room only by blowing the balloon.

The Metal Element works with the concepts of boundaries and touch. Here the children are not allowed to touch the balloon and have to use their breath, also a Metal quality, to move the balloon. It will become clear which children are very strong in the energy of rules and boundaries, making sure no one is touching their balloons, and which children are more flexible with boundaries and rules, touching and directing the ball with their hands! This stimulates Metal Element energy for all participating.

Water

The children lie on their stomach. The leader covers them completely with sheets of newspaper. The children are instructed not to move or make any sounds. When the leader gives a signal, the children are allowed to jump up and throw all the paper off.

Water Element exercises offer children the chance to be silent and still, and to experience the challenges that come with this task. It takes a lot of concentration for a child to be completely still and energy for patience to wait until being allowed to move into action.

These examples give an idea of how we create play exercises in the children's physical therapy clinic. In every session, we offer a game from each of the Elements to stimulate experiences that require the children to use skills, senses, movements, and behaviors that correspond with each of the particular Elements. All five of the Elements are offered in each session, and the games always follow in the natural cyclical order: Wood, to Fire, to Earth, to Metal, and finally to Water. The children are allowed to choose how long they want to play in each Element, and here we find that the children are naturally drawn to the Elements that are looking for the most stimulation to grow that day. Their inner network really guides them to what they need.

Another interesting outcome that we discovered when working with all Five Elements in the play groups was that the time with the group came to a natural close. The children somehow felt complete and ready to leave at the end of the last exercise. When the full circle of the Five Elements had a chance to be expressed, the ending of the cycle was felt by all.

To end this chapter we have included a whole section on the way the Five Elements can work in the many facets of the educational environment. These guidelines and examples can be integrated into any classroom setting or training program.

Teachers and Classroom Planning

Experience in the classroom setting has shown us the positive impact the cycle of the Five Elements can have on both students and teachers in the shared learning process. Whether planning a semester, day, specific period, or individual lesson plan, the natural flow of the Five Element sequence can be recognized and consciously used. All ages and topics can benefit and we have seen it implemented in settings from kindergarten through to high school, advanced academics, psycho-education, technical institutes, and movement classes.

When the natural cycle of the Five Elements is used in lessons plans or timed periods of a classroom day, a clear beginning and end can be achieved. We have observed classes where teachers and students demonstrated a spontaneous flow from Wood, to Fire, Earth, Metal, and Water that ended in a natural closure at the end of a lesson plan or activity. Somehow, all participants sensed without words when the sessions would end.

What the Five Elements offer in a classroom session is a natural internal and external order for new activities. This gives children a consistent pattern to follow, which allows them to experience security and develop a sense of their own inner order and rhythm. Children who do not have a sense of their own inner rhythm show signs of difficulty when given many choices for activities or put in unstructured classroom settings. Behaviors that would reflect this difficulty vary with age, but some early signs in elementary school children could include disruptive behavior when given open-ended choices, distracting other children, agitated body movements, withdrawal from classroom activities, defiance, aggressiveness toward other children, inability to make choices, and anxiety. These behavioral signs indicate that the open-ended activities or choices are too demanding for the child's senses.

Creating the external framework of the Five Element sequence in class activities can help children get in touch with themselves in the context of the group and focus of the classroom. For this framework to be effective, however, new opportunities to express the Five Elements should be presented continually. As creative and new activities are offered in the familiar Five Element sequence, a sense of security can be experienced, allowing more possibilities for a child to try new things and grow. This also allows room for recognition, acknowledgment, and respect for the individual children as they discover their unique expressions of the Five Elements.

Daily Classroom Structure with the Five Elements

At the start of the day or at the beginning of a new session, we offer a preparation stage. The preparation stage is a short exercise that allows the children to experience the Five Elements in an abbreviated form. This helps everyone to arrive, get in the mood for being at school or the next activity of the day, and begin to feel the flow of the Five Elements. We use the analogy of a seedling to describe the way the Five Elements support the learning process and students in the classroom.

WOOD

In the Wood Element stage of a class activity we want to prompt the development of the "seedling that will grow" during the session. Here we are dealing with the development of ideas, and then mobilizing the energy for creativity and movement within a child. In Wood Element activities we need to support children to work off surplus energy with gross movements and physical activity, and give them room to be creative while trying new activities.

FIRE

In the Fire Element stage of a class activity, our seedling reaches the flowering stage. Fire activities allow the children to engage with one another and experience the "all of us are in this together" feeling in the group as they learn a new activity—a Fire quality. Contact and communication with classmates, and opportunities for laughter and fun are necessities. Exercises in partners and small groups allow the needed group interaction for the Fire Element expressions.

EARTH

In the Earth Element stage of a class activity, our seedling bears its first fruits. In this phase of the cycle of the Elements, the students will become quieter and more focused. Exercises that allow the children to experience sharing while working on their own project should be used. This allows centering, concentration development, and being within oneself while feeling the common ground of everyone in the same activity. Continued support should be offered by the teacher, through repeating instructions, bringing the project "full circle" with visual/physical/verbal instruction and activities—strong focuses for the Earth Element. Sharing meals, serving one another, and receiving from each other promotes Earth Element stimulation.

METAL

In the Metal Element stage of a class activity, the fruit has ripened and the seeds have multiplied to be scattered by the autumn winds. In this phase, recognition, acknowledgment, acceptance, and respect, of both one another and the individual process, occur during the

208 CHILDREN AT THEIR BEST

session. An inner order is felt here as the student allows himself to be acknowledged in what he has accomplished and completed, or not. The teacher is mindful that he is the mirror for the student's self-esteem, self-value, and learning of who he is and what he is capable of at this time. If a student has difficulties with an exercise and becomes disruptive in the class, the teacher should offer acceptance with clear, non-shaming boundaries, to allow him to reflect on what he is struggling with in the learning process. Physical activities such as bowing, shaking hands, and creating space from one another to feel individual boundaries in the classroom are Metal activities. Acknowledgment in the form of rewards from the teacher is a Metal activity.

WATER

In the Water Element stage of a class activity, the new seed has found its place in the lap of the earth. It rests in the soil and contains all the information for a new cycle. Arriving at the Water Element stage is the final part of the session. Since the Water Element gives us the capacity for relaxation and regeneration, stillness and calmness are possible to introduce and what the students will gravitate toward if the other elements have been expressed insufficiently. In stillness we can listen to others; when calm we can wait until it is our turn and allow ourselves the relaxation we need.

Five Element Support for Teachers

Before we begin planning the session, it is helpful to prompt the flow of the Five Elements within oneself as a teacher. Each of the individual Elements can be stimulated with simple inquiry so that they are available to support all the functions needed when working with the class. In addition, you can try "Example 3: Opening the Gateways to the Five Elements and Clearing Your Head" from Chapter 13 to create your own mini-visualization of the Five Elements. You can be creative and use any of the Five Element examples in the following chapters to center yourself before beginning your day or a lesson.

Questions
WOOD

1. Do I have a clear picture of what I will be doing with the class in this session?

2. Is my plan consistent with a review of what we did last, what we are doing today, and what it will lead to for tomorrow?

3. Do I have a sense of what needs to move today with the students and for myself?

4. Am I prepared to allow for their creativity to come into the plan to support their learning?

FIRE

1. How will I engage the children in working together in this session so that they feel the purpose and comradeship of everyone learning the new materials today?

2. Do I have fun and laughter worked into the plan/lessons for today?

3. Do I feel my warmth and ability to connect with the children in an engaging way?

4. What will make this fun and joyful for me and them today?

5. Is my heart in the work today?

EARTH

1. Do I trust that I have enough ground under my feet to bring this new material to the children?

2. How centered do I feel in myself today?

3. What do I need to do to take care of myself today so that I am more available to take care of the needs of the students today?

4. What can I share today with the children that will feel nourishing, grounding, and centering to me and to them today?

METAL

1. What needs to be acknowledged for myself right now to move into this session/day?

2. What do I have set up for acknowledging the children's efforts and accomplishments today?

3. Are there any particular children who push my boundaries who I need to be clear with today and, if so, what is my plan to help them learn healthy boundaries in the classroom without shame, ridicule, or lowering their self-esteem?

4. What do I need in order to have clear boundaries today for myself and the children?

5. Do I feel my inspiration as a teacher right now and, if not, what do I need in order to do so?

6. Am I breathing fully and helping the children to breathe fully in this session/day?

WATER

1. How calm and relaxed do I feel in this moment?

2. Do I have any fears going into this classroom or session?

3. Is my listening open for what the children really need for today or this lesson?

Example for Integrating Five Elements into a Lesson Plan with Children

Once you feel you have your center, you can begin your session. Below is an example of a preparation stage exercise for a class, followed by a sample of a math session with an elementary school class.

Preparation stage

"Stand next to your seat and stretch up to the ceiling, as tall as you can. Imagine your feet are roots in the ground and stretch down into the ground at the same time! If you were a plant or a tree today, what kind of tree would you be? What kind of summer fruit would you make? Now turn to your partner and ask her what kind of tree or plant she is today, and if you can have a piece of her summer fruit. If she says yes, shake her limb or pick some fruit from her leaves. If she says no, say thank you anyway; next time maybe she will be ready to share. Now everyone hold hands in the circle and imagine that all the fruit and vegetables are put in the center. Lean to the left, lean to the right, and hum a sound that you make when you see something yummy in front of you. Imagine you take some of the fruit and eat it. Rub your tummy and stand with your hand on your belly. Take a deep breath with eyes closed and exhale. Now turn to your partner and shake their hand, thank them for the yummy fruit today, and go back to your seats. Sit with your eyes closed and feel the seat underneath your bottom. Feel how strong it feels and how it supports you. Say to yourself, 'I am ready to learn something new.' Open your eyes and get your pencils and math sheets out. We are ready to begin!"

Math Lesson Example

We begin with the Wood Element in the cycle. The Wood Element activity for the math lesson would first review briefly what the children remember from the last session, then present the new information, and show what it will look like when they are finished. It will offer something visual and with movement for counting or an example of what the math equation is doing. Fire Element activity will allow questions and clear communication for responses— reminding the children it is new, that everyone is working on the new problem, and encouraging them to keep trying and be courageous. Setting up an activity where the children are working in small groups or with partners with the new material is appropriate here. Engage in fun ways, not making the task too difficult, while allowing the children to feel whatever is arising. Accept the challenges they experience with warmth. The Earth Element will allow the children to bring the new exercise to fruition, completing some problems together as a group or by themselves, with a review on the board for the class to see. The Metal Element will be the acknowledging part where the teacher can offer acknowledgment for their efforts individually and offer some verbal or visual reward for showing or turning in what they have worked on. Some teachers let children move circles of success on a board, or on a sheet on their desk. This way they feel some inner accomplishment and the teacher can acknowledge them with a signature and/or encouragement for what they can continue to work on the next day. Making sure the children's efforts are acknowledged and respected is a strong focus here. Even if a child has been disruptive here in Metal, the teacher can acknowledge it was a rough day or session and make it better the next day with some suggestions for how to follow up with the student so that he does not feel incomplete or shamed, but is given awareness of the boundary of appropriate activity. In Water, the child puts everything away as the activity is finished and is given a choice to move to a quiet part of the room that has reading, drawing, or building activities. Continuing to do what they are doing quietly so the other children can finish their work is important; this also allows the lesson to settle in their system so that they can feel the completion of the Five Element cycle.

Conclusion

Playful work with children in the Five Elements can be created in many ways and in many settings. Children's furniture can be arranged and created to stimulate the Five Element senses; seasonal activities or various stations in the classroom could even be set up for children to play in all of the Five Elements. The possibilities are as numerous as you wish to make them because every activity can be associated with the Five Elements. More ideas are given in later chapters. Whether the examples are about professional settings or homes, any combination can be used when staying in the sequence of the Five Element exercises and games for children.

CHAPTER 11

The Role of Adults in Five Element Work

A Partnership with Children

Whether parent, teacher, therapist, or mentor, the role of an adult in Five Element work with children is one in which trust and acceptance of the developmental process must arise. Children need adults in their life who can listen to where they are, give guidance that allows them to discover and learn for themselves, accept their feelings regardless of how irrational they may seem and offer support that respects what they are capable of developing at this time. All of this is possible when the Five Elements have the opportunity to express themselves through us as adults when working with children.

When we get stuck in judging children, and start to view their feelings, behaviors, and reactions to be "wrong," we fail to support their growing process. We are struggling in our own capacity to manifest some of the more open levels of the Five Element expressions.

To really work from the Five Element perspective with children we have to remember that the aspects and qualities of the Five Elements we are observing in their development cannot be viewed as isolated energies that exist only within the child. Everything the child interacts with, which includes the adults in their lives, adds elemental influences that can affect their development. The way in which adults interact and direct children from the Five Element perspective is a key component to its success.

The Five Elements are present in our lives and can be seen in everything we do. As we begin to observe and assess the Five Elements and the ways in which they influence the development of a child, we cannot separate ourselves from the observation process. The environment that affects the children affects us; the activities that we direct to offer them stimulation in the Elements also stimulate our Elements. We unconsciously and naturally set up our personal living and working environments to support what our own developed Five Elements need to function. Now it is time to observe how our own Five Elements are expressed and see what other possibilities can arise as we begin to support children and their developmental needs.

This chapter asks you to reflect on how you have unconsciously learned to express the Five Elements as you interact with children. Reflecting on the ways our Five Element expressions respond to situations, individuals, and settings gives us the chance to be aware of where we come from as we interact with children. This awareness allows us to step outside of our personal space of reacting to the environment and into an observer role where we can see ourselves as a key component of the Five Element experience. When we begin to recognize our own Five Elements in our Five Element work with children, we can become a real guide and navigator for the children in their own elemental development.

The ways in which we have learned to express the Five Elements have come from our own early childhood experiences. As we work with children, we often come up against our own stagnation and impeded areas of expression. This is a natural part of working with the Five Elements and children. A wonderful aspect of this process, however, is that the more we work with children to prompt the flow of the Five Elements, the more their movement will open us. We cannot work with the cycle of the Five Elements without it influencing our own cycle, which means we too will experience new expressions of the Five Elements.

The Five Elements sustain us in a very specific way in our roles as parent, teacher, therapist, or mentor. Whether we work with children, adults, parents, or mixed groups, the Five Elements support us and offer us ways to work with others. The following descriptions and questions give a summary of how the Five Elements can arise for you as an adult working with children. Use them to reflect on your experiences and see what areas are naturally present and what areas you may have difficulty in finding expressions.

Five Elements Expressions in Adults that Support Working with Children
Water

The Water Element gives us a calm reserve to be in moments and situations when unknowing and confusion may arise. It offers us a capacity to be with silence, stillness, powerful outbursts, and strong reactions, and to have a deep inner trust that is supported by a depth and knowledge that a movement will come to help guide our work with children. The Water Element gives us the ability to listen to all of a child's responses to the activities, and to recognize that there is important information in what a child is *not* responding to or expressing directly in his behavior and style of movement. The Water Element allows us to feel a flow from one Element to the next, and to know when to move into action or be still. It allows us to know when to be silent and when to speak, when to support and when not to support, when to make boundaries clear and when to allow children to discover their own boundaries. The Water Element offers us the possibility of relaxing and flowing in the whole environment with children. Fear and anxiety are the red flags for reassessing what unknown factors are present that are making us feel uneasy about a situation.

QUESTIONS

1. How do you feel and respond when you are in confusing situations and don't know what to do?

2. What kinds of situations bring up uneasiness, fear, or anxiety when working with children? How do you respond in these moments?

3. How do you respond to situations that are new and unfamiliar to you when working with children?

4. What kinds of environments are difficult for you to relax in when you are with children?

5. What kinds of environments are the easiest for you to relax in when you are with children?

6. In your work with children, are there moments when you don't know what to do? If yes, what types of situations create this feeling, and how do you react?

7. What is your greatest fear when working with children?

8. What makes you feel the most calm and trusting when you are working with children?

9. What types of situations make you feel powerful when working with children?

10. What types of situations make you feel powerless when working with children?

11. How do you respond to children when they are expressing fear, uneasiness, or anxiety?

12. How do you respond to children when they don't know what to do in certain situations when you sense what needs to be done?

Wood

The Wood Element supports our ability to navigate through all of our work with children. It gives us our ability to see the multifaceted levels of what is happening with a child and what needs to be done for growth to occur. The Wood Element opens up the creative process, allowing us to envision a direction and image to move towards as we work with a child. It gives us the capacity to direct, lead, and select appropriate games, exercises, styles of movement, and situations that will help children to develop their ability to express all five of the Elements. A crystal-clear capacity to make distinctions between the past, present, and future is one of the gifts of the Wood Element. This allows us to see the big picture of a situation, which can give room for flexibility as we have the capacity to navigate through possible difficulties further down the road. Wood allows us to make clear decisions, so that all the details that need to be carried out for the creation of a developmentally supportive space can be planned. Frustration and anger are the red flags for reassessing our ability to see a child for who they are in the moment and what they are actually capable of expressing, as well as for a reassessment of our own capacities while working with children.

QUESTIONS

1. What kinds of situations make you the most angry or frustrated when working with children?

2. How do you express your anger or frustration with children?

3. What is your ideal dream or vision of how you would like to be as an individual working with children? What qualities, assets, and ways of being do you aspire towards?

4. Describe yourself as a parent, teacher, therapist, or mentor today. Is this different from the way you have been in the past or would like to be in the future?

5. How easy is it for you to see where a child is in this moment and to make distinctions between the past and future projections of what you would like them to be capable of?

6. How flexible or rigid are you when working with children? Describe a few situations in which you reacted flexibly or rigidly.

7. How is your creativity expressed when working with children?

8. How does personal growth and movement arise for you when working with children?

9. What types of environment make it easy or difficult for you to lead and direct children?

10. What kind of room do you give children to move, jump, laugh, or shout in your working or living environment?

11. How much room do you give children to be involved in the decisions and creative planning of their work, time, space design, and activities with you?

12. What do you experience when children get angry and how do you respond?

Fire

The Fire Element supports us in our ability to provide warmth and loving kindness in our work with children. With Fire comes a level of unconditional warmth that invites children to express the feelings and excitement that are present in the moment. This Element supports the relationship between the adult and the child or group of children working together. It enables us to create a feeling of togetherness in a group and to build the feeling of partnership throughout the whole experience. With Fire, the leader can create a sense of camaraderie, which shows itself as a warm, open-heartedness toward everyone in the group. Good communication skills and the ability to interpret for everyone what is happening in group activities are part of the harmonious expression of the Fire Element. We recognize the presence of the Fire Element when laughter, joy, and a lightheartedness with the children, the work, and the self arise. It has a vitality and energetic way of being present that allows us to feel connected to everyone in the room. A lack of openness to others' emotions and a heavy-hearted feeling are the red flags to reassess what is closing the heart and dampening the light warmth that the Fire Element offers while working with children.

QUESTIONS

1. What kinds of environment allow you to feel open to express yourself when working with children?

2. When do you experience the most joy and lightheartedness with children?

3. What makes you feel warm and connected to a child or group of children?

4. How do you create a sense of camaraderie between children when working with a group?

5. How open are you to the expression of emotions and feelings when you are working with children?

6. How would you describe your relationship to the child or children you are working with at this time?

7. Is it easy for you to communicate with children? When is communication difficult, and when is it easy?

8. What is your communication like when you are in a difficult situation with a child or group of children?

9. What does your heart want from your work with children?

10. Do you have fun when you work with children?

11. Describe a situation in which a cold atmosphere developed and a loss of contact arose when working with children. How did you feel then, and how did you react?

Earth

The Earth Element allows us to create the ground for all of the other Elements to express themselves while working with children. It is the energy that supports all of the processes, standing tall and steady like a Maypole as the Five Elements dance around playing in their unique aspects and characteristics. It provides us with the capacity to root ourselves firmly in our own knowledge, opinions, visions, and insights, while still supporting others' experiences that may differ. This allows us to stay centered and focused on what the children really need to be nurtured and nourished in their developmental process. It also gives the adult in the space a sense of being solid and grounded, capable of supplying whatever the children need in the moment.

Just as the earth naturally follows a rhythm from one season to the next, so too the Earth Element gives us the capacity to sense the rhythm of the Five Elements as they move from one to the other. This allows us to think logically and follow the cycle of the Five Elements as we support the movement of the exercises, games, and overall flow of the activities and experiences in the group. It reminds us of the common ground that we share with the children through this fundamental rhythm, and from this arises a sincere empathy and compassion for the struggles the children go through in their development. With this perspective, we are able to create a space that feels nurturing and unconditional in its ability to hold whatever expressions come into the environment when working with children.

The overall sense provided by the Earth Element is one of security—feeling that we also are supported, provided for, held, and capable of nurturing ourselves as well as the children in our lives. When we are unable to hold our own ground and focus on what is needed for the children we are working with, it is time to reassess what is missing in the support of the Five Elements for ourselves.

QUESTIONS

1. What is needed in the environment for you to feel grounded when working with children?

2. How steady and rooted do you remain in your own opinion, views, or insights when challenged by a child or another adult? What do you experience when this happens?

3. What types of activity do you do to create a sense of common ground between you and a child you are working with or among a group of children working together?

4. What is needed in the environment for you to feel centered and focused while working with children?

5. What types of things in an environment or situation create a loss of focus or centeredness when working with children?

6. What makes you feel supported in your work with children?

THE ROLE OF ADULTS IN FIVE ELEMENT WORK

7. Describe an incident in which you felt yourself unsupported when working with children. How did you react, and what did you feel?

8. How do you create a supportive atmosphere for children to play, work, and develop?

9. What makes you feel grounded when working with children?

10. How do you nurture yourself or take care of yourself when working with children?

11. How do you support children in learning how to take care of others and themselves?

12. How do you respond to children who are extremely clingy and needy, or just never seem to be able to get enough attention?

Metal

The Metal Element enables us to respect and accept all human beings as individuals expressing their own developed and undeveloped ranges of the Five Elements. This allows us to step outside the boundaries and expectations placed on children through traditional medical diagnosis and treatment plans, and hold a broad perspective and container for them to grow and experience the world so that they can learn clearer expressions of the Five Elements in their lives. Gifts of the Metal Element are discipline that offers new experiences to learn from (as opposed to punishment); boundaries that offer children room to sense themselves, others, and the space in between; acknowledgment of accomplishments and areas that need growth; and objective observations that support mirroring for self-awareness and positive self-esteem. These capacities are possible because of the innate sense of timing and clear boundaries for self and others that the Metal Element provides.

Metal Element energy enables us to accept and recognize the expressions and reactions of children because of the awareness of personal boundaries and limitations each child has in her development. This discernment of limitations is also extended into the environment and perception of self as the participating and leading adult in the Five Element space. The Metal Element gives us the capacity to create the rules, boundaries, and disciplinary action if needed. These arise out of a respect for and acknowledgment of the learning process that is in motion, without harsh blaming, shaming, or making any of the children feel that they are wrong in their explorations. The Metal Element makes us open to the inspiration that the Elements offer us when the cycle of the Fundamental Rhythm of Life is allowed to flow, and enables us to feel a deep connection to the developmental process we are facilitating.

When we experience harsh judgments, blame, or shame, and are incapable of creating clear rules and boundaries from a respectful space, then it is time to reassess how acknowledgment, acceptance, and respect are being presented in our own life and how this is influencing the way we are working with children.

QUESTIONS

1. How do you create your own space and self-boundaries when working with children?

2. What are your boundaries in terms of time, contact, and behavior with the children in your working or living environment? How do you define these boundaries with children?

3. What kinds of boundaries exist in the physical environment that you work or share with children? How do you define these boundaries with children?

4. How do you express respect for the children in your working and living environment?

5. Is respect expressed by the children in your working and living environment? If so, how is it expressed?

6. What kinds of behavior do the children elicit that leave you feeling not respected? How do you respond in those moments?

7. How easy is it for you to let go of disturbing experiences that you have had with children, and to create space for new possibilities?

8. What situations or experiences in your work with children are the hardest to let go?

9. What helps you to resolve these disturbing experiences with children?

10. Are there ways in which you feel you would like to be more accepting of children's experiences and behaviors? What would you need to let go of in order for that acceptance to be present?

11. How easy is it for you to develop awareness of the personal boundaries of the children with whom you work?

12. Are these boundaries respected? If yes, in what way?

13. How do you respond to children who do not seem to have a sense of personal boundaries and space around them?

14. How do you respond to a child who is fighting, blaming, or being disrespectful to other children or yourself?

15. How do you make your boundaries for yourself, and how do you make the space clear to the children you are working with?

16. List a few experiences that have given a sense of acknowledgment, acceptance, and inspiration to you and the children with whom you are working.

Adults as Companions in the Five Element Space

For the authors of this book, the most meaningful part of the process of working with children in the Five Elements is the joint creation and participation of the dance of the Five Elements. As adults, this is a constant process of becoming aware, of witnessing, creating, and participating in the different forms of the expressions of the Five

Elements. This means that our role as adults in the Five Element space is not the conventional "role of the therapist" that is often more distanced from the activities of children in various types of play groups and therapy. Instead, it is a natural playful dance that allows one to be a companion as well as a leader in this guiding, therapeutic space.

Our role in the Five Element playing field is that of a navigator on a joint voyage in the cycle of the Five Elements. We are the conductor for the environment and the caretaker of the space, offering activities that give room for all of the Elements to be expressed. All the activities and changes to the environment that we guide are manifestations of an innate, ancient cycle. As the children get to play in the range of the activities offered, they have the chance to increase their capacities to express themselves. The adult becomes a partner for the children, piloting them through a space that offers them the potential to express all their innate possibilities of being.

In contrast to the children, we adults perceive this unfolding process at a rather mental and descriptive level. A child will experience each Element much more naturally, because the patterns of the Five Elements are still in development and pre-cognitive. Yet both adults and children can gain the essence of this experience when the energy of the Elements moves in the cycle. We are all dancing on common ground that is directed by the Fundamental Rhythm of Life. We too have the possibility to expand our awareness and expression of who we are in this world.

CHAPTER 12

Creating Five Element Environments for Children

This chapter is a compilation of suggestions for adults to begin finding ways to introduce the Five Elements into their personal lives and into the environments of the children they are working with. There are a few principles to remember about working with the Five Elements from this perspective which we want to review before beginning.

The first thing to remember is that all five of the Elements are observed and used each time we work with a child. After going through the questionnaires in the various chapters, you might think, "I know exactly which Element my child has imbalances in," and then assume that you only need to work with the exercises for the Element revealing the most imbalances. Our experience has shown us that working with only one Element is not the most successful way to offer children the opportunity to grow out of difficult patterns and imbalances.

> All five of the Elements are observed and used each time we work with a child.

When one Element is stagnant and finding difficulty in its ability to develop and express itself, all of the Elements are affected. This is because the Five Elements are truly a cycle: each one supports the movement and development of the next, and counter-balances the expression of another in a cyclical pattern. The continued flow and expression of all Elements reveals our personal Fundamental Rhythm of Life. We have all gone through difficult times in our lives when we have experienced what it feels like to be out of balance or, in our words, when that fundamental rhythm has lost its timing.

> When one Element is stagnant and finding difficulty in its ability to develop and express itself, all of the Elements are affected.

When all of the Five Elements are available for children to play with in the environment through games, activities, and exercises, children are naturally drawn to whatever types of movement and stimulation they need to grow. They may spend more time playing in one Element than the others, but all five are still needed to make the experience round, giving the child the opportunity to express all of the Elements with the new stimulation just experienced.

> When all of the Five Elements are available for children to play with in the environment through games, activities, and exercises, children are naturally drawn to whatever types of movement and stimulation they need to grow.

Creating the Five Elements in the Child's Physical Environment

We will approach this chapter in four ways—a child's bedroom, the home, the classroom, and the therapy room—listing ways in which to introduce the Five Elements into the lives of children through various aspects of the physical environment.

We invite you to experiment with these ideas. Go back to the chapters on the Elements and review what the characteristics are for each of them. Find the expressions of the Elements in yourself and play with the ideas and exercises to discover what they feel like and how they can bring a sense of harmony and inner balance. A strong emphasis on a single Element is possible to help support a child with constitutional weaknesses in one of the Elements, while still making sure that all the Elements are expressed in the different environments for overall development. We welcome you again to the cycle of the Five Elements.

A Child's Bedroom

WOOD

The key to supporting the development and balance of the Wood Element in a child through her room is to find age-appropriate furniture, toys, exercises, and props that support the expression of large movements, discovery, creativity, and noise. The following are some suggestions and correspondences that can help offer this.

- *Colors:* Use different shades of green. Paint the walls green, create a floral scene with trees or a jungle, or use fabric for bed linen and window treatments that has a lot of green in it.

- *Furniture:* Large pezzi ball, small indoor scooter, or small tricycle; large mat on the floor with space for tumbling; children's furniture that has strength for climbing or creating tunnels and forts.

- *Art center:* An area set up for drawing, coloring, or age-appropriate children's crafts.

- *Older children:* Teens and older children still need some space for movement. Pezzi balls for sitting on at the desk, a mat to stretch, dance, yoga, doing martial arts, and an indoor hoop and basketball can be helpful. Also, visual art such as holograms, puzzles, pioneer or survival computer games, and art materials.

FIRE

The key to supporting the development and balance of the Fire Element in a child through his room is to find things that express what the child loves and is enthusiastic, joyful, and passionate about.

- *Colors:* Hues of reds are great for bringing the stimulation of the Fire Element into a room.

- *Passions:* If a child is passionate about sports, dance, animals, a Disney character, actor, or singer, having pictures and representations of what they really enjoy in life is important. Calendars, posters, themed bed linen, stuffed animals—all of these are great ways to support and give expression to the things a child feels connected to.

- *Pictures:* Photographs of friends, family, pets—people and animals with whom they have a strong, warm, and loving relationship can be very supportive for Fire Element balance.

- *Relationship items:* Sometimes children form bonds with inanimate objects such as a blanket, a stuffed animal, or a truck—whatever the child's imagination has created to make something real and has developed a relationship with. These items need to be accepted as important and connected to the child's heart at this time in his life, and given a place in the child's room.

- *Furniture:* The furniture should have a playful and fun appeal.

- *Laughter:* What makes this child laugh? Objects or pictures that bring giggling and laughter into the child's room is a great support for Fire Element development.

EARTH

The key to supporting the development and balance of the Earth Element in a child through her room is to find things that help her to feel at home, centered, supported, held, and balanced. Also include things which help the child to express her nurturing side. Musical instruments, drums, play tents, and teepees are Earth Element expressions and supports.

- *Colors:* Yellow and gold give expression to the Earth Element.

- *Canopy or four-poster bed with sheer curtains:* Hanging sheer fabric from a four-poster bed or hanging a ring with a sheer canopy over a bed can create a soothing, comfortable feeling of being held and cradled for children.

- *Nurturing center:* Having a doll house, space for baby dolls with cribs, a pet center area with stuffed animals, or homes for insects, reptiles, or other real or imaginary pets is important for a child to develop the nurturing aspects of the Earth Element.

- *Play kitchens, restaurants:* A play center with make-believe kitchen, food, dishes, and restaurant.

- *Plants and window garden:* A small window garden for a child to grow flowers or herbs from seedlings.

- *Bedding:* Soft, full, fluffy bedspreads, pillows, or stuffed animals that the child can bury herself in and snuggle into at night.

- *Consistency:* Keeping the room the same and consistent may be important for a child who shows a lot of imbalances in Earth Element development.

METAL

The key to supporting the development and balance of the Metal Element in a child through his room is to find ways to support the creation of his own order, organization, private space, and rules.

- *Colors:* White is the color for the Metal Element, and stainless steel and silver can also be used to support the expression of Metal.

- *Space:* The overall space of the room of a child with a lot of Metal imbalances can be extremely helpful for his development. The room should feel that it has space in it, and should be orderly and organized, and tidy and clean, as if everything has a purpose and is utilized; even the empty space in between can feel as though it is part of the organization and has some value.

- *Patterns and simplicity:* The simpler the color schemes and patterns, the better. This room needs to look uncluttered, with clear, sharp, and distinct lines and patterns.

- *Furniture:* Straight lines, not rounded and curved, possibly painted white, or more modern metal-framed furniture can be very supportive for Metal Element energy.

- *Self-expression:* The child's wishes, visions, ideas for organization, and color choices need to be included and respected for Metal Element development.

WATER

The key to supporting the development and balance of the Water Element in a child through her room is to create a space that makes her feel calm and looks inviting to relax, be quiet, and rest.

- *Colors:* Blue and black are the colors that can bring a sense of calm into a room.

- *Still space:* Creating a space that looks inviting to come and sit down and be silent gives expression to the Water Element— for example, corner with a cozy chair, or a beanbag chair close to books or facing a window to sit and gaze out at nature.

- *Lighting:* The room needs to be able to be darkened for proper rest, and lighting should be as close to natural light as possible; fluorescent lighting can sometimes create a very fast irritating flicker or sound that can make it difficult to rest.

- *Sound:* Be aware if a child's room is next to a laundry room or bathroom in a house. The constant sound of machines or running water through pipes can be disturbing and make it difficult for a child to rest.

- *Art/posters/decorations:* Soft watercolors, murals of clouds, blue ceilings, and gentle nature scenes of water can all bring a sense of the Water Element.

- *Comfortable, soothing bed:* The bed should look as if it invites the child to rest and sleep.

Home Settings

There is room for a lot of creativity and flexibility when setting up your home to support the expression of the Five Elements for your children. You have many rooms to play with and can create whatever kind of space and time you want to offer your children by way of activities, tools, and visual stimulation for the Five Element expressions. Read through our suggestions and go back to the chapters on the individual Elements if you need more information to spark your own creativity and ideas. No one knows your children like you do, so create what will work for them and their personal desires and development. Have fun!

WOOD

For the Wood Element to develop, children need room to move, shout, scream, jump, be creative and imaginative, and express their bursting, growing energy. This will, of course, vary with age, and the physical environment can change as their developmental needs shift—even adults need room to move physically and express their creativity. Parents need to look at how much room they give their children to express all of these qualities in the home setting, and look at some of the following ideas for offering more possibilities for the Wood Element expressions if needed.

- *Rooms:* You can set a room up in your house that has space and permission to be a play room that allows shouting, running, jumping, building, drawing, and painting. A "yes" space is very supportive to the Wood Element. Giving children that room to act out and stretch their limbs and branches grows a healthy tree.

- *Furniture:* Age-appropriate furniture that allows jumping, bouncing, rolling, and tumbling can be a great support to Wood Element development. Try to have the family's main living space filled with furniture that you don't have to worry about so that your children have room to express what naturally wants to come out of them.

- *Room to move and tumble:* Open space with as little furniture as possible or furniture that can easily be moved, such as beanbag chairs, is a great support for Wood.

- *Colors:* Variations of greens.

- *Toys and games:* Small indoor vehicles, such as a low-riding tricycle or a truck that is strong enough to sit on the back—toys that they can ride on through the halls if the house is big enough; rocking horses, small exercise trampolines, indoor nerf basketball with hoop, indoor balls, pogo stick, moon shoes, pezzi balls—toys that allow movement and coordination.

- *Games:* All kinds of sports, Sharks and Minnows, Red Rover, creativity that allows leading, directing, and decision making.

- *Offering choices:* Offering your children choices whenever possible allows the decision-making process of the Wood Element to develop. Clothing, meal planning, sport activities, play dates with other children, and choosing gifts for friends and family members are all examples of daily choices that parents can offer children.

- *Leadership games:* Giving children free time with friends to create their own games that they can lead or follow is also very supportive to the Wood Element.

- *Pioneer/discoverer/explorer/protector:* All of these roles in games in physical activities can be supportive.

FIRE

Laughter, joy, expression of emotions, warmth, communication, relating, open-heartedness, relationships, partnerships, openness— all of these are expressions of the Fire Element that can support the development of children when present in the home.

- *Colors:* Reds and pinks stimulate the Fire Element.

- *Fun, warm rooms:* Rooms with colors that look fun and inviting are great for the Fire Element. A warm feeling can be generated by family photos, children's art, candles, fireplaces, cozy furniture, and small gifts and sculptures given and created by your children.

- *Enabling communication:* Finding ways to enable your children to express their emotions, thoughts, and feelings is important. Examples would be a feeling chart, where a child can place velcro features on to a face to express an emotion, or rituals at the dinner table for family members to share their "high" and "low" experiences for the day—anything that gives room for everyone to share, including the parents, so that children can learn to express what they have experienced and are experiencing in their life.

- *Activities and games in the home:* Games, exercises, activities, and tools that offer children the opportunity to come together as a group, to feel a connection and partnership with one another, and to be able to communicate clearly and feel a sense of warmth and relationship within the family will help the development of the Fire Element. Charades, birthday parties, tag, Red Rover, board games that foster communication, playing house, and so on...

EARTH

The home itself is the center of the Earth Element expressions. It is where a child returns at the end of the day and where much of the development of feeling at home within the self develops. The home setting needs to offer a sense of nurturing, groundedness, safety, unconditional holding, and support. Being able to digest our physical nutrition and life experiences are Earth Element qualities, and, when developed, they allow one to feel content and round in life.

- *Colors:* Yellows and golds will support Earth Element expressions.

- *Nutrition and meals:* Balanced meals, consistent eating schedules, and focus on the food during meal times (without the distraction of TV or books) are important for Earth

Element development. The digestion is supported best in a child when they are allowed to eat at a comfortable pace and without distractions or other forms of stimulation.

- *Cooking together and planning meals together:* Baking, working with dough, cooking meals, and participating in meal preparations are all supportive activities for the Earth Element.

- *Gardening, plants, or growing herbs:* Working and digging in the soil, planting seeds, and harvesting fruits, vegetables, and herbs are all Earth Element activities that ground a child.

- *Swings/rockers/hammocks:* These are great sources of stimulation for the Earth Element—furniture that allows a child to feel their center and be supported.

- *Old-fashioned handicrafts:* Knitting, crocheting, pottery, macramé, and beading are all examples of old handicrafts that support Earth Element development.

- *Caretaking with pets:* Participating in the nurturing and caretaking activities of pets in the house is supportive for Earth Element development.

- *Activities and games in the home:* Games, exercises, activities, tools, and props that allow children to find their balance, feel what is under their feet and sense the ground, or experience supporting, helping, cooperating, and working together on a common goal with others—all of these support the development of the Earth Element in children.

METAL

The home setting is where the initial values in life are learned. Sacred values, respect, inner and outer structures of the self, self-discipline, awareness of personal boundaries and the boundaries of others, and our relationship to organization and cleanliness—all of these are qualities of the Metal Element that are introduced in the early home environment of a child.

- *Colors:* Whites and clean, crisp lines in patterns and designs are stimulants for the Metal Element.

- *Organization:* Creating an organized house where the family functioning has a system and order is very supportive for Metal Element development with children. Rooms designated for different activities, laundry, cleaning, eating, papers and finances, specific areas for homework, backpacks, lunchboxes, shoes, relaxation—all of these create external organization and stimulation for children which affects Metal Element development.

- *Schedules:* Schedules create order, rhythm, and respectful boundaries for children that allow them to feel the space of time in themselves, the world, and in their family lives. The Metal Element supports the whole body and our ability to function in the world. Consistent meal times, bed times, play time, and work/school schedules help a child to experience a rhythm in life and begin to feel their bodies in relation to the activities of life.

- *Cleanliness:* A certain level of cleanliness in a home is part of a routine that can teach respectful boundaries for self and other objects and people.

- *Respect:* Learning to treat others as you would like to be treated is part of Metal Element development. Respectful communication and examples with other people and with objects is supportive to Metal Element development in children.

- *Boundaries:* Learning boundaries in the home, with clear teaching and age-appropriate expectations, supports the development of the Metal Element in a child. Accepting innocence and offering children opportunities to learn about boundaries in the environment fosters self-knowing and awareness which is part of the development of boundaries in children.

- *Acknowledgments:* Recognizing and acknowledging children's achievements big and small fosters self-awareness which is part of Metal Element development in children as they learn their boundaries.

- *Responsibilities:* Offering opportunities for children to have age-appropriate responsibilities with household activities supports the development of Metal.

- *Activities and games in the home:* Games, exercises, activities, tools, and props that allow children to have physical contact with others, to experience the physical boundaries of themselves and others, or to find respect and acceptance—all of these support the development of the Metal Element in children.

WATER

For the Water Element to develop, children need room and time to relax in life. The home setting is often filled with the hustle and bustle of the twenty-first century. Finding time to slow down, listen, feel the depths of self, and be with the unknowns in life is important for the development of Water Element expressions in a child.

- *Colors:* Blues, blacks, and calming colors contribute to Water Element stimulation in a home.

- *Quiet, restful spots:* Areas that invite places to sit down and observe nature, read a book, and relax on a bench outside or in a bay window are all invitations for Water Element activities.

- *Rituals:* Family rituals that are passed down from generation to generation carry depth and meaning that is part of the Water Element energy and supportive for children to experience and get in touch with their Water Element.

- *Lighting:* Areas in the house that offer dim lighting and relaxation are supportive for Water.

- *Reading at night:* Reading to children at night before bedtime or naptime is a Water Element activity that allows children to slow their day down and experience a quieter pace within themselves.

- *Rest and relaxation:* Acknowledging the importance of rest and relaxation, and creating space for this in a family, supports the Water Element development in children.

- *Activities and games in the home:* Games, exercises, activities, tools, and props that allow children to face their fears, experience a level of trust, to relax and be still, or going inside to feel— all of these support the development of Water Element expressions.

School or Classroom Environments
WOOD

Finding ways for a classroom to support the expression of the Wood Element can be challenging since movement is one of the primary ways children develop in this Element. Nevertheless, an area is needed in which children are allowed to move throughout the day as well as visual and experiential items that spark creativity, discovery, and planning skills.

- *Colors:* Various colors of green.

- *Free movement/play corner or station:* Some teachers create a space where they allow children to go to once their work assignments are completed. This area typically gives children the choice to play on the floor or a table, or sink into a beanbag, and has toys such as cars, dolls, Lego, books, art paper and crayons, or any number of items that allow a child to choose and create imaginary games on their own. Just having permission to get up and move and allow the mind to create freely can support Wood Element development in a classroom setting.

- *Art and sculptures:* Pictures of children's art and famous artists from all over the world, rotated and changed throughout the school year, can be a great stimulus for Wood Element expressions.

- *Games and activities:* Games that foster leadership, creativity, problem solving, and following are developmental stimulants for the Wood Element.

FIRE

A classroom can support the expression of the Fire Element through visual aids that express relationships, joy, humor, communication, and emotional learning. To find a way to make a room look fun and enjoyable to spend time in is important for the Fire Element and children's development.

- *Colors:* Reds and pinks are the colors of the Fire Element and can be used to decorate in the room in many ways.

- *Humor/fun:* Expressing humor in a classroom can be great for the Fire Element—for example, a corner on the blackboard with a joke for each day/week, funny pictures that are rotated and displayed for the children to interpret and communicate what they find funny, or a fun corner with some kind of stimulus for the children to be lighthearted and joyful during the day.

- *Props that express emotions:* Pictures that show people experiencing an emotion and a caption asking "What are they feeling?" or a feelings chart where the children can put a velcro face to express the way they are feeling today under their name on a wall—anything that gives children a way to understand emotions and communicate them.

- *Visual aids:* Pictures that express relationships, hugs, warmth, and partnerships between children and adults. Joyful pictures, fun colors, and pictures of children laughing with others and relating to animals, people, and things in a warm, joyful way all can stimulate Fire Element expressions.

- *Games and activities:* Games that create partnership in the classrooms are a Fire Element stimulation. Creating a sense of partnership and common purpose is especially helpful in large classrooms. The question to ask yourself as a teacher is:

"Are you a dictator or a leading comrade?" Pulling the class together as a group in a joint, team-like partnership with one another can be very supportive for the development of Fire Element expressions in children.

EARTH

A classroom can support the expression of the Earth Element by including things that create the sense of common ground and nurturing for the children. Consistency in the environment creates security, which is also important for the Earth Element. Overall, the classroom needs to give children the experience of being supported, with outlets for nurturing activities with classroom pets, for baking, and for activities that help children develop a balanced sense of self in relationship to everyone around them.

- *Colors:* Yellow and gold will support Earth Element expressions.

- *Cooking station:* Something that we all share is cooking and eating, and this nourishes the development of the Earth Element. Even if the room is not set up with a kitchen, a crock-pot, bread maker, or a cutting board and bowls can be great resources for making simple meals and snacks together. Dough that can be pounded and shaped is also helpful.

- *Music:* Dance, melody, and rhythm all support the development of the Earth Element and are simple things that can be added to a room for children to experience.

- *Pet/doll corner:* Having dolls and stuffed animals to create nurturing games is very supportive for the Earth Element. Live animals in the classroom, which the children learn to feed, water, touch, and care for, can also be excellent tools for Earth Element development.

- *Gardening and clay:* Planting, digging, and growing in a garden or having potted plants in a classroom are great supports for Earth Element development in children. Clay and playdough can also stimulate the grounding activity of the Earth Element.

- *Individual support:* Finding a way to support each child individually within a classroom can be challenging, but it is very important for some children to feel grounded and secure in the school environment.

METAL

A classroom can support the expression of the Metal Element through structures and systems that create respectful boundaries for the classroom environment and each other. A classroom that has a way of acknowledging successes and uses disciplinary actions that provide learning opportunities rather than punishment when boundaries are not respected also fosters Metal Element development.

- *Colors:* White is the color for the Metal Element.

- *Organizational systems:* Visual organization with as little clutter as possible can be very supportive to the Metal Element in a classroom. If there are systems for stations, tasks, arts and crafts, building centers, and math and reading areas, which are clear and age-appropriate for levels of responsibility, Metal Element development can find support.

- *Respect:* Having visual aids and examples of diversity—for example, different cultures, different foods, different art— and having discussion that includes respecting differences are very supportive to the development of Metal. Rules that have respectful consequences that allow learning and new respectful actions to be experienced foster the presence of Metal in the environment.

- *Defining boundaries:* Finding ways for children to recognize their own personal boundaries and understand the boundaries of others and objects is a very important part of the development of the Metal Element. The distance of the chairs from each other, the sharing of classroom supplies, placement of individual backpacks and coats, individual cubbies—all of these things need to be thought out carefully in terms of placement and rules, and then presented to the children so that they can learn how to respect the personal boundaries of other people and their belongings.

- *Fair, clear, consistent rules:* Consequences that are fair, consistent, respectful, and lacking in condemning or judgmental qualities are very important for the development of Metal Element expressions and should be posted and reviewed before used within the classroom setting.

WATER

The Water Element can be expressed in the classroom environment through creating activities and physical spaces that allow rest and relaxation.

- *Colors:* Blues and blacks.

- *Relaxing, quiet area:* Many elementary school classrooms have a reading area set aside with a bookshelf full of books and comfortable chairs or beanbags for children to sit down and read. Depending on their age, children sometimes also need room to lie down and rest while they read or take a break from the activity of the day. This is becoming a rare setting in public schools and is something to consider when there are students who appear to become hyperactive or lose a sense of their boundaries when they are over-stimulated or tired from classroom activities. Some children exhibit reactive behaviors because they are tired and there is nowhere for them to stop and let the mind and body rest away from activities and other children. Finding comfortable furniture for the children to relax in—a beanbag chair or two, a plush square of carpet with pillows to lean on, anything that is child-oriented for relaxation—is supportive to Water Element development and can change the whole dynamics of a difficult classroom.

- *Listening center:* An audio center with headphones and recordings of stories and music in a comfortable setting such as the reading area can be very supportive for the Water Element.

- *Calm, flowing schedule:* Creating a schedule that does not rush the children and can calmly flow from one project or subject to the next is very important for the development of the Water Element.

Occupational/Physical Therapy Room for Children

WOOD

Ways to encourage the presence of the Wood Element in the therapy room to support its expression in children include having room for the children to move, jump, shout, explore, and be creative in making up games and activities. Having an environment set up to stimulate gross motor skills and accommodate flexibility, movement, and tumbling with many different kinds of activities and ideas from the children is important.

- *Colors:* Colors of green stimulate Wood Element expressions.

- *Exercises and activities:* Games, exercises, activities, and tools that offer children large movements and the ability to plan, lead, and direct are important to stimulate the development of Wood Element expressions.

- *Self-reflection question for physical therapists and occupational therapists:* How flexible am I in allowing the children to create and direct their visions and ideas in the therapy room?

FIRE

Ways to encourage the presence of the Fire Element in the therapy room to support its expression in children include creating an environment that looks cheerful, fun, warm, and as if it has space for a lot of expressive activity.

- *Colors:* Reds and pinks stimulate Fire Element expressions.

- *Joyful pictures:* Fun colors, as well as pictures of children laughing with others and relating to animals, people, and things in a warm, joyful way, can stimulate Fire Element expressions.

- *Exercises and activities:* Games, exercises, activities, and tools that offer children the opportunity to come together as a group, to feel a connection and partnership with one another, to be able to communicate clearly, and to feel a sense of warmth and relationship to others will help the development of the Fire Element.

- *Self-reflection question for physical therapists and occupational therapists:* How do I provide warmth in the therapy room to develop playful partnership and connection between myself and the children or between the children in the groups I lead?

EARTH

Ways to encourage the presence of the Earth Element in the therapy room to support its expression in children include offering a space that feels supportive, grounded, nurturing, and safe to express whatever is arising.

- *Colors:* Yellow and gold will support Earth Element expressions.

- *Exercises and activities:* Games, exercises, activities, tools, and props that allow children to find their balance, feel what is under their feet and sense the ground, and experience supporting, helping, cooperating, and working together on a common goal with others will support the development of the Earth Element in children.

- *Self-reflection question for physical therapists and occupational therapists:* How do I create a space of unconditional holding, so that the child/children feel grounded and supported to find their center and balance in life?

METAL

Ways to encourage the presence of the Metal Element in the therapy room to support its expression in children include creating a space that has safe boundaries, that is organized, orderly, and tidy, and where everything has its respected place and can be returned to that place when finished being played with or used. Also, creating an atmosphere that holds a deep respect for the children and the work that occurs in the room, and of acceptance of who they are in this moment and what they are capable of, is an important expression of the Metal Element that will support their development in the therapy room.

- *Colors:* White is the color of the Metal Element and is often used on the walls or ceiling since true acceptance and respect are a strong part of the foundation and boundaries being created with children in Five Element work.

- *Exercises and activities:* Games, exercises, activities, tools, and props that allow children to have physical contact with others, to experience the physical boundaries of themselves and others, and to find respect and acceptance support the development of the Metal Element in children.

- *Self-reflection questions for physical therapists and occupational therapists:* How do I create an environment that fosters the development of respectful inner and outer boundaries in children while still allowing them to experience new dimensions of themselves and others? Do I allow children to express in this moment what they are capable of doing and being?

WATER

Ways to encourage the presence of the Water Element in the therapy room to support its expression in children include creating a space that is easy to relax in, comfortable, friendly, and not scary or intimidating in any way. Even creating a specific area that is inviting as a quiet spot, where children can be silent and sit if they want to, can be a big support for Water Element expression in the therapy room.

- *Colors:* Blues and blacks. Blue ceilings with clouds painted on them can be very calming, or one wall in the room could have a similar mural.

- *Water:* The sound of water in a small waterfall, a fish tank, or even toys that look as if they have water in them which can be picked up and played with can support the Water Element.

- *Exercises and activities:* Games, exercises, activities, tools, and props that allow children to listen, relax, or activate the proprioceptive system will support the development of the Water Element.

- *Self-reflection questions for physical therapists and occupational therapists:* How relaxed and at ease am I with the children in the therapy room? How relaxing is the environment for children and their families in my therapy space?

CHAPTER 13

Ideas, Exercises, and Examples from Practice

This chapter is a compilation of ideas, exercises, and examples that form the foundation of our work and message. When we step into the Five Elements and their work, a new range of exploration is available that opens creativity and invites everyone involved to experience genuine expressions and growth in themselves. The ideas and exercises in this chapter come not just from our own daily practice, but also from those who have taken the work out into the field and experimented with the way the Five Elements move them to work with others in personal settings.

We will begin with exercises that can be applied to adults to stimulate the Five Elements, and then offer examples in different age groups and settings for children. It is important to remember that these are *ideas* and *examples* of exercises. You are invited to use them for inspiration and to add on, change, or recreate these ideas in other applications with the Five Elements or to create brand-new exercises to suit your needs.

Examples of Exercises for Adults

Example 1: A Short Five Element Fantasy/Visualization

Ask your group to find a comfortable seated position in which they will be resting for the next ten minutes. When ready, ask them to close their eyes and take five deep breaths, making the exhales longer than the inhales.

Notice where the tension is in your body that keeps you from breathing fully. Put your hand on that place on your chest, abdomen, shoulder, or neck, and imagine now as you breathe in that your body is filling with air to push back on your hand; as you exhale, your hand sinks deeper into the area, dissolving the tension. Do this as many times as you need to feel the relaxation of your body; breathe in and out until you are comfortable in your chair.

Give the room a couple of minutes to relax.

Now that you are relaxed, allow yourself to go to a memory of a safe, relaxing scene. Find a place to sit or lie down in the scene, and imagine you can feel the temperature of the air as you breathe, the ground underneath you, and the serenity of the setting. Close your eyes in this safe place, and feel yourself drifting into a deeper relaxed and calm state... With your eyes closed, you hear a gentle wind behind you and you turn to see what is there. As your eyes open, you see that you are in the middle of a beautiful, luminous, deep, azure-blue pavilion. The air around you is the perfect temperature as it swirls in rich hues of blue and black. It feels like water in a current as it flows through you, and you feel it carry you deeper and deeper into total relaxation. The pavilion has a voice and it says to you, "I am the Element of Water within you. Through me you can find deep peace, relaxation, and rejuvenation. Feel the flow and movement of me in you. I give you the power and energy to flow and adapt in all situations in life. I give the relaxation in the unknown and the reserve to endure all experiences. In me comes a trust of the depth within you and it is in me that you find rest and peace from the outer movement in life. Close your eyes again and feel my power, gentleness, and constant presence." You close your eyes in the blue pavilion again and feel the power and gracefulness of the Water Element moving through your whole body.

Again the wind rustles around you, and the air feels fresher with a certain aliveness. Curious, you open your eyes in this serene scene and see that this time you are surrounded by luminous green lights in a brilliant green pavilion entwined in spring-green vines and blooming flowers. The freshness of the scene makes you feel like stretching and moving. So you stretch your body from head to toe and feel the urge to move even more. Ideas of projects that you have wanted to complete or are working on start to come into your mind with an energy of excitement and newness. A voice from the green pavilion speaks: "Welcome to the green pavilion of the Wood Element. Here, all of your visions in life can be made clear. Clarity of what exists in the moment, dreams for new possibilities in the future, and recognition of what has existed in the past are all available to you here. Feel the power and desire to stretch, grow, and expand in every direction."

Again, the wind rustles before your eyes and you feel a surge of energy move upward with a lightness as the light changes from green to luminous shades of red. You hear laughter as if something is tickled by your fascination with what is changing in front of you as the wind and swirling colors calm down and you find yourself in a brilliant red pavilion. It is warm, the sun is shining, and there are birds flitting around with one another and communicating across the branches. Something feels extraordinary in the way the warmth of the sun shimmers and everything feels connected and dependent on the other for the balance before your eyes. The wind blows the branches, the birds dance on the flow, and the sun shimmers sparkles from everything around. The scene is light, cheerful, deeply warming, and touching to the heart, as if everything in the pavilion has purpose and intention in each movement. The sound of laughter earlier now has a voice and speaks to you, saying: "Welcome to the red pavilion of the Fire Element. Here, your heart can relax, feel the lightness of life, the connectedness to all that is, and the way everything brings a balance and peace to the heart. True communication and joy comes from this space. Feel the lightness of your heart, and feel what your heart wants to express in life."

You close your eyes once again, feeling a joy and fullness in your heart with the warmth of the sun on your skin. The wind begins to rustle again and you know without opening your eyes that the pavilion is changing once more, transitioning to another phase. You feel a contentment in the process and a solidness of the ground underneath your body. Slowly opening your eyes, you see hues of earth tones in yellows, golds, oranges, and clay reds. The pavilion has transitioned to a harvest gathering with barrels of pumpkins, fruits, seeds, and grains bountiful around the edges of the luminescence shining into the darkness. It is a harvest waiting to be distributed. "But to where?" you find yourself asking. "Wherever it is needed," responds a voice to the question. "Now, now," says another voice, "they need more explanation than that." "Welcome to the golden pavilion of the Earth Element," says the first voice. "We are here to make sure everything gets nourished in life," adds the second voice. "Including you," adds the first voice. "And everything around you that you take care of," says the second voice. "It's really not as confusing as we are making it sound," says the first voice again. "The Earth Element gives you a ground underneath your feet to always stand on, a place to rest at night, and nourishment on all levels to satisfy your appetite. In the golden pavilion you come home to yourself, and that takes a lot of solid ground under your feet and a balance of taking care of your needs and the needs of others and obligations in life." "Well spoken," says the second voice to the first. "Thank you," responds the first voice. "So what do you need to feel like you are home inside yourself?" the two voices say in unison as the wind starts to swirl again...

Feeling yourself reflecting on the last question, you take a deep breath and close your eyes again, knowing the pattern and signs of the transition now. The air gets cooler and crisp, and this time you are surrounded by a white luminous light. A voice from the light says, "Welcome to the white pavilion of the Metal Element. Take a deep breath in and feel the boundary of your lungs, and then exhale, feeling the release and letting go of the air from your body. What happens next? You will breathe in again, and out again. Feel the rhythm that happens in your body naturally, without even thinking about it. Every breath you take has to let go for the next to come in. This is the Metal Element in your life. Your internal and external rhythm of letting go of stages of life, of old thoughts and old patterns, makes room for the new to come in. This pavilion is guided from the inspiration of your heart, and carries that inspiration out into your life. All personal boundaries are supported, created, let go of, and recreated here in this white pavilion. The most important things that are needed to sustain life remains, and those that are not are let go of. So breathe in this white light and feel the connection to everything through the air, through time, through the passing of generations, and into the next generations to come."

The wind swirls again and you find yourself in the original safe space and scene you started at. You stretch, breathe, feel your body once again in the room, and, when ready, open your eyes and sit up. Please exchange with another person in the room something you want to share from your experience with the Five Element journey.

Example 2: A Five-Minute Visualization for Centering

This visualization can be used before walking into a meeting, a presentation, or before entering into a project you need to get done. It can be done while sitting and waiting for a child to get out of school, upon waking before starting the day, or in an office on a coffee break. The Five Elements offer us the ability to quickly come to our center and have self-awareness of our weaknesses and strengths, and offer support for the areas we know we need to work on. Adapt the language of the visualization to meet your individual situation or general observation of life, and only use the questions which come to mind that apply to what you need at the moment when repeating the visualization.

Water: We always start with a deep breath, allowing our exhale to become longer than our inhale, and we do this until we feel a physical calmness and awareness of our breath moving in and out. Imagine you are like a strand of kelp in the ocean, allowing the current to sway your body and joints, feeling the power, gentleness, and continuous movement of the water around you and through you. When you feel relaxed in the flow, ask yourself: "Is there anything creating some fear or anxiety right now in my life/in this situation? Are there factors I don't know about that I am not looking at right now? What do I need to listen to in this situation? What do I need to hear? What fluidity is needed in my life or this situation? How can I bring relaxation, calmness, ease, steadiness, and power into my life/this situation?"

Wood: Imagine you come out of the water and in front of you is a forest full of trees. You see a tree that you are attracted to and imagine yourself inside that tree, as if you are the tree. Imagine the strength and desire of the roots reaching down into the warm, thawing earth, your branches itching with excitement to stretch with the new buds for growth on your branches, and your trunk in the middle feeling strong and balanced with your growth happening in every direction. You breathe and imagine your life like the tree and the tasks you are trying to accomplish right now in your life. Ask yourself: "What is my plan? Did I finish what I needed to do last? Can I delegate some of what is left or put it on a list for later?" Clear the plan for what needs to be completed with a plan for how to complete it. See the vision of what you need to do next. How far can you plan ahead? Sense if the future plan gets too far away from the steps in between. Step back, trace the steps of what the plan is now, and how far it can go. Feel a strength from your torso to support the plan and what you can create right now for stability and the future.

Fire: Take a deep breath again, and ask yourself: "What is joyful in my life right now? How am I expressing my joy? Is there too much focus on this, or too little, in my life? Do I dream about it, or actually take action to do joyful activities? What creates lightness, laughter, a sense of community, and partnership for me in my life?" Take a deep breath and remember a scene from your life that was light, joyful, playful, and full of laughter. Remember something simple that you did to feel light and alive. Was it music, dancing, stretching, running, or singing? Feel this in your body. If you can do it after this visualization, do it; if not, make a plan for when you can. Think of a symbol, like a beautiful stone, a bird singing, or a friend or child smiling, and give yourself a way to recall this when you need it. And then ask yourself: "What is my communication like in my life/ situation right now? Does it hold an opening for connection, understanding, and warmth? Is there something that needs to be communicated clearly in life/this situation right now?"

Earth: Take a deep breath and feel the ground under your feet, the seat supporting your body, or the bed or ground under your body. Feel the way you can relax with its support, feeling yourself let go without worry or concern that it will hold you up. Ask yourself: "How am I supported in life or this situation? How am I supporting others in this situation? Where is my common ground in this situation or in life? Am I taking care of myself and others in this situation and in life? What is the balance of that activity? Is there anything that needs nurturing or holding in my life or in this situation? What do I need to create stable ground under my feet in my life or in this situation? What are my views and opinions in life or this situation, and do I feel strong enough on my own to hold the ground and compassion for others in theirs?"

Metal: Breathing deeply again, ask yourself: "What needs to be acknowledged with respect in my life or in this situation? What do I need to sort out in life? What is most valuable in my life or this situation that I want to have take shape?" Still breathing deeply, acknowledge your own value and the value of your experiences in life, and those of anyone else in your life or the situation you are in right now. Take another deep breath and allow yourself to remember an occasion where you felt a sense of oneness with everything. Maybe it was watching a sunset, or sitting on the side of a mountain, or watching the rhythm of the ocean surf going in and out... Recall a moment when you felt a contentment and connection to nature and everything around you. From this space, ask yourself: "Is there anything that I need to reflect on in my life or this situation right now? What are the boundaries between me and the world or others in this situation? How can I hold respectful boundaries and awareness of myself and everyone in my life right now? What is the most valuable thing I want from this moment in life?"

Example 3: Opening the Gateways to the Five Elements and Clearing Your Head

As described in Chapter 2, particular emotions are associated with each Element. In Japanese medicine, they are referred to as "gateways" to the world.

Probably everyone is familiar with the feeling of their eyes being not yet fully open in the morning, or of having had "a bellyful" ("I don't want to see or hear anymore!"). In this series of exercises, the gateways are cleared and our outlook on the world is opened. Here is the sequence for a group (and it's just as suitable for an individual):

- Find a place that you like in the room, and stand with your feet shoulder-width apart.

- Shake your hands and arms fully, to loosen up.

- Then bring the palms of your hands together in front of your chest, with your fingertips pointing towards the ceiling. Press your palms together. Maintain the pressure for a few breaths and then release. Repeat twice.

- Now rub your palms vigorously together to activate the *Ki*. You'll start to feel a sensation of warmth.

- Slowly move your hands apart and place them on your back, in the kidney area, and rub there hard, until you get a sensation of warmth.

- Slowly let your hands drop. Bring your palms together once more in front of your chest, and rub them until they are warm.

- Follow the next steps to open the *Ki* in the Five Elements to bring some clearing focus.

Opening the Gateways
EYES: WOOD ELEMENT
Now rest your middle fingers on your upper eyelids and your ring fingers on the lower lids with eyes closed; massage your eyes with gentle, slow pressure. If you wear contact lenses or if you don't like the feel of it, you can do the exercise without direct contact, by moving your fingers slowly back and forth in front of your eyes.

TONGUE: FIRE ELEMENT
With the tip of your tongue, make circles in the space between your lips and your teeth. Try it in both directions—often one way is easier than the other.

MOUTH: EARTH ELEMENT

Place the sides of your index fingers above and below your lips. Massage these areas by stroking in opposite directions with your fingers.

- *Head:* Massage your head, making little circles with the fingers of both hands. Don't forget the back of your head. Then take handfuls of hair in both hands and pull gently.

- *Face:* Rub your hands together again hard to make them warm, and then "wash" your face.

NOSE: METAL ELEMENT

Allow the hands to face each other with fingers resting together and pointing towards the ceiling. Place the balls of the thumbs on either side of your nose, with your fingertips pointing towards the ceiling. Slide the balls of your thumbs up to your forehead, and back down to the corners of the nose. Repeat several times.

EARS: WATER ELEMENT

Now lay your hands against your cheeks, with the index fingers behind your ears and the middle fingers in front of your ears. Massage the area behind and in front of your ears vigorously, with both fingers.

Centering and Completion

Bring your hands back down and let them rest below your belly button for a few breaths.

Example 4: A Parents' Evening—
Dealing with Difficult Topics

This example can be used to work with any group, ranging in age from older teens to adults, which is dealing with a difficult topic. This group example focuses on the issue of bullying in a school and a parents' meeting. The format works with inquiry through questions about each of the Five Elements, which are asked in the sequence of the cycle of the Elements. You can choose some of the questions or create your own, and do a series of evenings with the same format or one evening and pick one or two questions from the list. One

Element per evening could also be done, with a series of five to six meetings offering more time for planning and implementing programs for change.

Introduction and Activation Stage

A short visualization that walks the group through the Five Elements, or Example 3, which moves the energy in the Five Elements in the emotions, is recommended to bring everyone to a center in themselves and offer some relaxation around the tension on the topic to be worked with. After the Five Element exercise, present the focus for the group and whatever the events are that have led up to the evening being held. From this point, the group can be broken down into partners to inquire further from the Five Element perspective for one-evening events, or the group can discuss the questions as a whole. It is recommended to work with these questions before problem solving and implementing new rules, actions, and decisions. The following introduction could be used:

> We are here tonight to talk about what we have been experiencing at school with the increase in bullying between groups of children. Some of the parents here have children who have been bullied, and some are parents of children who you feel were unfairly disciplined as a result of the bullying incidents. We are going to break up into pairs to discuss this first from a series of questions that will help us to deepen our insight into the situation at hand. Take turns asking each of the questions in the five sections and then we will get back together to discuss what suggestions and ideas have arisen.

Questions
WOOD

1. What ideas or plan did you come with today?

2. What do you want to know or have made clear about what is happening here at the school with this situation?

3. Is there frustration or anger about this situation? If yes, talk about it.

4. Do you have a strong vision of what to do with this situation at school?

5. What do you think the students are angry about with this situation at the school?

6. What needs to grow and change in this situation at the school?

7. How do you see your role as a parent in helping to change this situation at the school?

FIRE

1. How did you first hear about this situation at the school and what was your reaction?

2. What do you want to communicate about this situation right now?

3. What has your communication been like with your child about this situation?

4. How is your heart impacted by this situation?

5. What will you communicate to your child after this meeting?

EARTH

1. What is the common ground of all the children here at this school and how do you see it being nurtured?

2. Describe what you think a school community should look like. What is missing from that vision in the school community right now?

3. How can the community support what is happening with the students in this situation at the school?

4. What kind of support and nurturing do you think the students need from the school to change this situation right now?

5. What kind of support and nurturing does your child need from home to help him or her with this situation?

METAL

1. Discuss your ideas about "respect" and how you think it should exist in a school setting.

2. Share what levels of respect you see happening and not happening in the school setting.

3. What models of respect have your children been exposed to?

4. Discuss how you see revenge or "social justice" being demonstrated in society today and the ways you think that affects the students. Also share your own feelings about revenge.

5. Share your own model of respectful boundaries with your student if comfortable.

6. How is acceptance and forgiveness modeled in our community and society?

7. What needs to be acknowledged about this situation at the school?

8. What ideas do you have about bringing more respect for individuality, acknowledgment, and acceptance of differences into the school setting?

WATER

1. What frightens you the most about this situation at school?

2. What are the biggest questions you have about this topic/situation?

3. What message is coming from the students in this situation that you think we may not be hearing?

4. How can we open our listening to the students about this situation?

5. Is there something that feels powerless/powerful for you as a parent in this topic, and if so, what is your reaction to feeling powerless or powerful?

6. Talk about how you see your own child feeling powerless or needing to feel he or she has power in school.

Example 5: Five Element Movement Group—A Project for Adults with Back and Posture Problems

This example describes a one-hour Five Element session conducted with a group of adults experiencing back problems and posture issues. This session could be applied to any adult group that is able to be physical, and the goal is to move the Five Element energy to open the mind, emotions, and/or physical ability of the group. Examples of groups could include: parents dealing with children with particular developmental issues; substance abuse groups; school parent groups; team-building for businesses; and college warm-up groups for young adults entering college. This group example consists of 12 participants and the course leader.

Materials Needed

Pezzi balls (exercise balls, 2 ft in diameter)—enough for half the number in the group plus three extra.

Introduction and Activation Stage

The participants stand in a line and form a circle facing the back of the person in front of them. Each participant taps the person in front of them on the back. They then take hold of the person's waist and all sit down together on the floor with legs extended out straight on either side of the person in front of them. Together, while still holding the waist of the person in front, the group leans forward and backward, and then does a side stretch toward the center of the circle, and then outward. Then they try to stand up together as a group.

Exercises
WOOD

Everyone stands in a circle, facing the center, to the accompaniment of very rhythmical music. Slowly, step by step, members of the group are instructed to begin to bring parts of their body into a dance. At first, only the head should move, while the rest of the body remains still. Next, the shoulders join in, along with the elbows and hands, and also the entire upper body. Now the hips can move, then the knees, and finally the feet. Now everyone is free to move as they please. Slowly, the group returns to stillness. Each person chooses a partner. One person will lead, running across the room with the partner following and trying to imitate the leader's movement. The imitating partner is instructed to stay aware of his own perceptions. Roles are then reversed. After the exercise, they can briefly discuss their experiences. To conclude, everyone runs across the room dynamically, with vigorous arm movement.

FIRE

The group divides into pairs, who stand opposite each other with a pezzi ball between them. Each pair tries to lift up the ball without using their hands, runs across the room without losing the ball, and then changes direction and goes back to the starting point. Next, both partners try to turn around at the same time without losing contact with the ball so that they end up back to back with the ball between them. Then two pairs meet and try to exchange the balls.

Next, with the partners sitting back to back on one ball, the group forms into a circle. Half of the group faces toward the center and the other half faces outwards. First, partners make their backs meet and begin rolling simultaneously back and forth, sometimes with smaller movements and sometimes with larger ones. Now the partners bob up and down together, trying to find the same rhythm on their ball. Next, the whole group tries to bob on the balls matching the same rhythm, using vocal help when needed. Now the fun begins: as the inner partners in the circle continue to bob upwards in the same rhythm, the outer partners in the circle try to move to the ball on the right, on command, changing balls and partners, while they try to keep the same rhythm going. This is repeated several times, and then the inner circle tries to do the same thing, with the outer circle keeping the rhythm and the bouncing consistent.

EARTH

Each participant in the group chooses a new partner or stays with the one they are already working with. One of the partners finds a stance that is balanced and comfortable. The other partner bends him gently in different postures while the feet of the standing partner stay in place. The standing partner slowly returns to the original position. This is repeated several times.

Both partners stand on one leg opposite each other, with arms extended and palms touching. Each tries to make the other lose balance.

METAL

All participants run across the room and try, while running, to perceive their breathing and the movement of the rib cage. Everyone now makes themselves quite large while inhaling and quite small while exhaling.

Everyone chooses a partner. One of the partners stands with eyes closed and tunes into how he is standing and how the space around them feels. The other partner approaches quietly and stops at a distance where he thinks the standing partner can sense him. The first partner then attempts to sense how far away the other has stopped. When he has an idea, he can open his eyes and compare. After reversing roles, the partners discuss their experiences, discussing the actual and imagined distances.

WATER

Gentle, relaxing music plays in the background. One of the two partners kneels down and lays her upper body across the pezzi ball. The other gently rocks her back and forth on the ball and then massages on her back and helps with stretches. Then the partners exchange positions.

Examples of Exercises for Children
Ages 5–7

The following are examples of exercises used with children in a variety settings that range from occupational/physical therapy clinics to classrooms, counseling practices, and homes. They can be used to inspire your own creativity for implementing the Five Elements with children you are working or living with.

Example 1: Florian—Individual Work with a Six-Year-Old
The Carrying Power of Earth

When Florian came to the children's clinic in Germany, he had just begun to attend first grade. At this point, the teacher was doubtful

IDEAS, EXERCISES, AND EXAMPLES FROM PRACTICE

and wanted Florian to leave the school, since he constantly disrupted the class. He could not sit still in a class to do projects or his work. He was always rushing from one activity to another, turning his attention to everything but the class. His disruptive behavior made the orderly progress of the class difficult for everyone else. His schoolmates shunned him on account of his aggressive demeanor. He struck out around him at the slightest provocation and he had no friends in the class.

At first, we put him into a group with five other children, three girls and two boys, all of the same age. He celebrated his entrance into the group when, in his words, he "really shook things up." Every time Florian entered the group room, something would go wrong, whether it was the thermostat, the cork floor coming loose, or the wall clock. The room had survived many children's groups for years, but whenever Florian entered each session, something would be disrupted.

Because of his exaggerated and rough way of making contact, he scared children off at first. Florian's manner and appearance brought out aversion and repulsion in almost everyone with whom he came into contact. His loud and dominating behavior rang out through the practice like his vigorous insults, and everyone knew: Florian was there!

When the children were busy with a group activity, such as building something, Florian's blossoming fantasy found expression in describing some violent and bloodthirsty horror scene. When the others didn't go along, he insulted them and disturbed their playing for so long that nothing else happened. He always had to take over the starring role, and could do everything better, faster, and higher. When someone came too close, he immediately became aggressive and struck out.

Numerous attempts to converse with the mother failed. She never came to parents' nights and missed scheduled appointments. Florian regularly came late to sessions (he was regularly brought too late for the session), so that we never saw the mother face to face. We only spoke with her once. At that time, it became apparent that Florian could watch whatever horror movies and videos he wanted at home, since this would occupy him so he wasn't a burden for his mother. After this conversation, it was clear to us that we could not expect much support from this side.

The breakthrough for us came one day in the group when we had worked with a big swinging cloth that we hang in the room. Everyone was sitting in this cloth, which looks like a giant oversize hammock, and swinging. Florian's movements became ever wilder, and the cloth swung almost to the ceiling. All the children began to clamor and rejoice at the swinging movement, and each time the cloth neared the ceiling Florian stuck his torso over the edge, and pretended he was going to jump. We were left gasping! One of the girls from the group suddenly tried to hold Florian, and said to him, "Please, don't do that! I'm scared for you!"

All at once Florian was startled. He climbed down from the cloth and sat quietly in a corner. His face was all soft, and he was mumbling to himself. "She was scared for me. There's someone who is scared for me!" His eyes were filled with tears.

At this moment, it was clear that the Earth Element gesture of being cared for touched Florian and we knew then what we needed to do to really support the continued work with him. We took Florian out of the group and worked with him on his own. We concentrated on making sure Florian was offered as much Earth Element stimulation as he needed in the Five Element exercise each session. Our attention was focused on strengthening the Earth Element and watching for the signs of naturally balanced Earth expressions developing in him.

For us, as Five Element therapists, it was fundamentally important to make our own expressions of Earth appear clearly and be perceptible, and to let go of all feelings of aversion and rejection based on our earlier experiences with Florian (which was not an easy thing to do!). We offered him the Earth Element in the form of a protected "space," which had a container or sense of home with walls. We encouraged him to use the whole space and feel the space in the room we provided, accepting that he could move and find his ground in the whole space offered. He was allowed to discover how big this space was, and what it felt like to occupy the space fully.

Every session thus needed a great deal of structure and distinct exercises that worked in each of the Five Elements. It was also important to make sure the full cycle of the Five Elements was completed each time. Florian also needed a great deal of sincerity, respect, and compassion from the therapist, to give him the chance to create trust.

We also made certain that all activities or actions Florian started in the session were completed and had a chance to come "full circle" in him before starting anything new. The motion, activity, or exercise was carried through to the end once it was started. With this focus, he was increasingly able to endure a moment of pausing, a particular quality of Earth, before he took on something new.

Very cautiously, we brought an atmosphere of caring into the session: the encircling, carrying element of Earth. As a "big boy," he avoided snuggling or physical closeness, yet this need became more distinct as his Earth began to express itself. For this, we invited him into our big sitting bag and wrapped him up snugly, or let him climb into a thick wool blanket that was gathered at the top and suspended from a rope attached to the ceiling. We would swing him with very gentle movements. After a session, he emerged all sweaty but very calm and turned inward.

Soon Florian began to bring little presents for his partner in the session: a cake, an Easter egg, or a flower. In the next session we worked with clay. At first, we made prints of hands and feet, before proceeding to make rounder shapes. There were balls of every variety, and Florian seemed to like the feeling of smoothness and roundness. From one particularly beautiful ball, he made a candle holder, which he took, together with a candle, as a present for his mother.

Another session emphasized rhythm (the rhythm of the earth). We drummed with large African conga drums, and then continued the rhythm first with our feet, then with our whole bodies.

The main focus of another session was on the center, balance, and solidity. At the heart of this were balance exercises, such as working with a pezzi ball or standing on one leg and trying to push each other over. Balance activities of all kinds belong here: one partner sits down and feels her stomach, while the other shouts nonsense or makes unexpected noises. During all of this, she must not make a face, while she continues to feel her stomach.

Although we stressed one aspect of the Earth Element in each session, it was extremely important that the therapist herself made the Earth Element appear through her behavior. We express this inner adjustment in the following sentences, spoken only to ourselves:

"It doesn't matter what you do, I know you are worth caring for."

"I like you despite all the hard corners and edges."

"You get unconditional support from me during this session."

"I have great respect for your efforts and your struggles to find balance."

After a few sessions, the Water Element could be brought more and more into play, whether through a relaxing story or when Florian listened to a piece of music while rolled up in the sitting bag, or when he was given a little foot massage. He was also able to listen to others, accept other points of view, and make his own ideas known through discussion. He began to be able to wait until it was his turn. Soon, Florian was ready to return to the group to try out his newly discovered abilities and behavior patterns. Of course, it is desirable to convince parents to work with us, for many of the ideas mentioned above can be integrated into home life and create support—in this case the Earth Element—for everyone.

Example 2: Mom and Me—A Mother–Child Project with First and Second Graders

This example is a session we conducted in a mother–child group within the framework of a ten-week elementary school project. Weekly meetings lasted 75 minutes. Ten mothers and their children and two Five Element therapists were present. Children attended either first or second grade. Participation in this project was voluntary and in addition to classroom instruction. All Five Elements were presented at each meeting to support the full cycle for the mothers and the children.

Environment and Materials Needed

One large, empty room (classroom size), one large cloth (e.g. a parachute tarp that is almost as large as the room), one thick rope (at least 1 inch thick and 4–5 yards long), tennis balls or physical therapy "hedgehog balls," 11 x 14 inch painting paper, and paints or crayons. All participants should be comfortably dressed and wearing nonslip socks or gym shoes.

Introduction and Activation Stage

After the pictures were drawn we began with a tapping massage on the arms, legs, stomach and back, which was repeated every week.

TAPPING MASSAGE

Making a loose fist with a loose wrist, we start at the chest and tap down the arm to the palm where we clap the hands and then take the loose fist up the back of the arm and to the shoulder; repeat on the opposite arm, three times on both sides. With loose fists tap down the front of the legs to the feet, and then up the inside of the legs. Tap down the sides of the legs to the feet, and then up the inside of the legs. Tap down the backs of the legs to the feet and then up again on the inside of the legs. Repeat again three times. Using the finger tips, tap the face and then the top, back and sides of the head. Stretch tall to the ceiling with arms in the air, and then relax forward while bending over and allow the arms to shake like a rag doll. Stretch arms to the ceiling again and stretch to the left, and then become the rag doll again, and repeat stretching to the other side and become the rag doll once again. End with closing the eyes and putting both hands on the belly to breathe and feel one's center.

Everyone does their own tapping massage. This stimulates the flow of energy, activating the metabolism, making contact with self, and bringing oneself present to the room.

Exercises

WOOD

The mothers and children walk around the room vigorously, swinging their arms loosely and in exaggerated motions. After some minutes of loosening up with this, they are called into a circle facing the center, and the group members are instructed to start moving their body, one part at a time. They start with the head only, moving it as they wish, feeling the movement of the head from the neck; next, the shoulders, arms, torso, and hips, and finally the legs and feet. It is important to add one body part at a time and allow them to feel the individual muscles and limbs, developing body awareness. Music can be added to give more freedom and for the group to get a feeling for movement.

The effect of this activity is to stimulate body awareness, planning of movement, orientation in the room, expressive movement, and coordination.

FIRE

Everyone is instructed to run around the room. The parachute tarp is spread out in the room, and two children are chosen for the exercise first. Child A gets under the cloth, while child B gets on top. The remaining members of the group spread out around the tarp and grab hold of it. The group lifts the tarp and makes big waves while child B tries to catch child A who is running around somewhere underneath the tarp. This creates a lot of laughter. After the roles are reversed, children who want a turn are allowed to go next. Then the whole group takes hold of the parachute tarp and they swing it together back and forth. At a spoken signal, everyone releases the tarp.

This activity stimulates the ability for contact, and encourages laughing with one another, having fun, and creating a sense of "together we are strong."

EARTH

Everyone is instructed to go around the room on all fours and is asked to feel how the earth supports and carries them. Everyone picks a partner. Partner A "bends" partner B into different positions. Then B comes slowly back into a centered posture, and the roles are reversed. Finally, both partners stand on one leg opposite one another. They hold hands and each then tries to make the other lose balance.

This activity stimulates the ability for everyone to find their center, solidity, and standpoint.

METAL

The mothers and children walk through the room again and are instructed to be aware of their breathing and the movement of their rib cage.

The long, thick rope is placed on the ground in a circle. The mothers and children are instructed to all get inside the circle. Different kinds of movement and position are suggested, such as going on all fours, walking in squat positions, or making a motions with the arms. As the group does these motions, the leaders make the rope smaller and smaller, instructing them to be aware of the space between them and to try to not touch each other as the space gets smaller and smaller.

This activity stimulates social competence, self-perception, respect for one's own boundaries and those of others, acceptance, and tolerance.

WATER

The group moves throughout the room. The rope is removed and the group is asked to move freely throughout the room again. Tennis or hedgehog balls are rolled out into the room, and quiet, relaxing music is played.

Participants pair off. One of each pair lies on their stomach while the other massages the neck, shoulders, back, and legs with the hedgehog ball.

This activity stimulates the ability for courage to allow something new, readiness to accept situations, coming in contact with one's own depths, and relaxing.

Observations of this Example

The pictures drawn at the beginning of this project were used to help us to observe their personal situations on the basis of the Five Elements. We have selected four of these, which are reproduced below. Unfortunately, no pictures were painted as a follow-up to the project, and this would be recommended to offer more individual feedback with the children. What is striking about these pictures is the representation of the physical form—for example, the lack of feet, arms, or hands; arms and legs that are only present as bumps; and the absence of the mother despite the specificity of the topic.

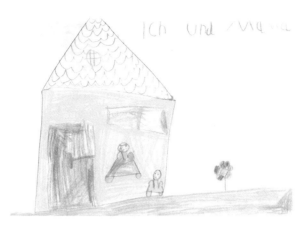

In this first picture, the arms and legs are depicted only as bumps. Mother and child are at home. During the exercise sessions, this child exhibited conspicuous problems with perception of the body and coordination. It was as if his limbs simply hung from his body without having a particular function.

ich und MAM
A

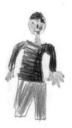

In this picture, titled "Me and Mom," there is no mother to be seen (and during this project the mother was often not present). Furthermore, we see distinctly formed hands, but no feet. The mother is the initial ground a child "stands" on in his development and for mirroring, connection, and nurturing support as he develops in the world. Healthy bonding and attachment with a consistent relationship is important for stable Earth Element characteristics to develop. The lack of awareness of feet in this picture reveals a level of ungroundedness and undeveloped awareness of the feet/ground that this child stands on. We do not really know what creates that, so further inquiry with the family would be needed to assess the developmental stage this child is representing and an inquiry with the intention to support the family to help the child find balance, as opposed to analytical judgment or pointing out faults.

The boy further expressed this lack in Earth Element development during sessions, when he would move constantly throughout the room, without finding a spot where he could settle down. He could only find his place within the group when one of the leaders took him by the arm, seated him on the ground, and stayed with him. From this protected standpoint, he could watch events and participate internally. His whole body was soft and supple then. This "big strong boy," as he was otherwise, gathered the power of the Earth Element with this support from the leader and the group.

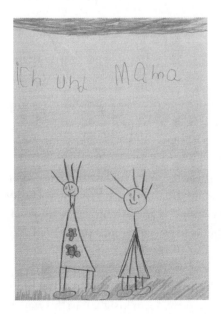

Here the head sits atop a long neck and is thus in a position to keep an "overall point of view." The figures stand on solid ground with powerful legs. The image lacks arms and hands, which makes action possible for a child.

During the project, this boy showed great enthusiasm for all mental tasks—in particular a great ability for math, which came to the foreground once. Otherwise, he kept himself in the background and had great difficulty participating in the group movements and events. He was unaccustomed to using his arms and hands.

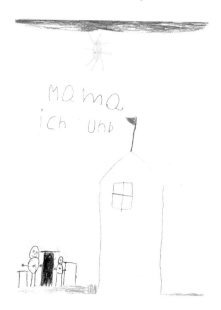

This child still lacks a precise conception of his/her body, and perception of space is also poorly developed, as depicted in the picture above with the relationship between the adult person and the table.

During the project, this child exhibited a particular form of the Wood Element, which was very pronounced on the one hand (aggression and temper), yet insufficiently developed on the other hand, with respect to the perception of his/her body.

Through the use of pictures that the children paint before and after a project, the leader can gain important signals about the changes in children through the course of the project. As we have seen, such pictures provide an insight into the way the Five Elements are being expressed in the children's perceptions of their body, relationships with the participants, and their self-awareness. This can offer more information to support children in the Five Element exercises offered and give some record of progress if pictures are drawn at intermittent times throughout the 10 weeks.

Example 3: A Kindergarten Project—"Playing in Japanese" (Ages 4–5) by Andrea Weidenfeller and Nina Behrens, Baby and Child Shiatsu Therapists

In the Nibelungen Kindergarten in Heppenheim, a Five Element project was carried out on the theme of "A Trip to Japan." Thirteen children aged four to five years old participated. The objective was to "travel" through all the Elements during this session. This was the children's first experience of working with the Element theme.

Materials Needed

- a pen

- adhesive labels

- a ball

- tennis balls

- poles

- large gym mats or padded floor covering

- crates

- wall bars

- carpet tiles

- wooden clothes pins

- a long bench

- beanbags

- clear, plastic painters' drop cloth

Introduction

The following introduction enables the children to get to know one another and tune into the topic. All the children sit in a circle and roll a ball to each other. When a child gets the ball, she says her name, and it is written down on a sticky label and stuck on her shirt; then she rolls the ball on to the next child. The name labels are intended for the activity leaders, so that they can address the children by name during the session.

The Five Element Game Begins

While still in the circle, the teacher asks, "Who knows something about Japan?" Ask around the circle whether anyone knows something about the country. Gather the children's ideas. A few examples of questions for prompting:

- Who's traveled by airplane before?

- How long did the flight take?

- How long do you guess it takes to fly to Japan?

"Today we are going to go to Japan and cross the big sea!"

Journey Across the Big Sea to Japan—Wood

A photo like the one below is printed on an 8 x 11 inch piece of paper, laminated, and stuck on the wall for the children to see during each of these exercises.

Wood Element Exercise: Tennis balls and poles are placed underneath big gym mats, which causes the mats to move like a "jelly floor."

The aim for the children in this exercise is to be creative, try something new, and be flexible (the moving foundation). The children individually have to try to cross "the big sea." (For example, to begin with, the children try to walk upright, and then creep or crawl; some of them might mime swimming movements.)

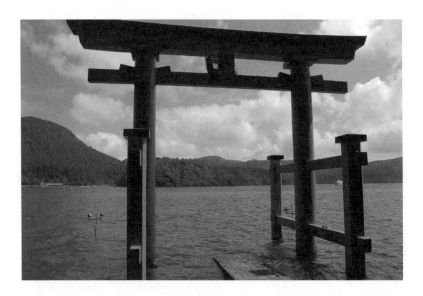

Crossing Mount Fuji—Wood

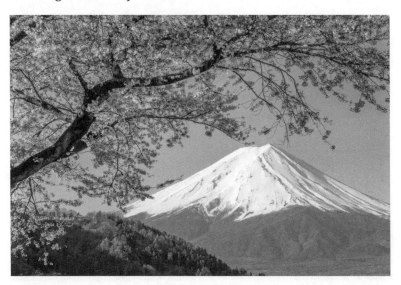

Wood Element Exercise: Crates and objects that are varied in height are set up one after the other in a row. An "ascent" is constructed in front of wall bars, and after it the "descent." In this way a "trail" is created, representing Mount Fuji.

The children scramble up and over the crates, clamber sideways along the bars, and climb back down on the other side.

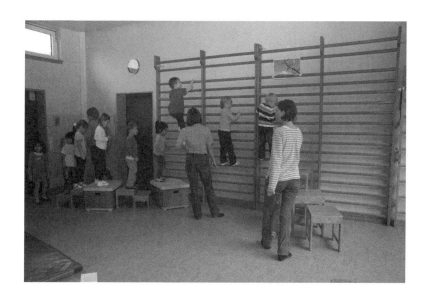

The Way into Town—Wood to Fire

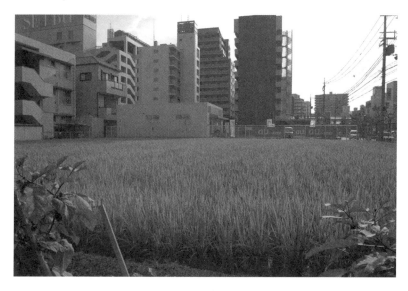

Transition from Wood to Fire: In pairs, the children make a team and set off on the way into town. In addition, they have to cover a certain distance with a "wheelbarrow."

The child behind holds the feet of the child in front and lifts them up. The child in front walks on his hands like a "wheelbarrow." The path (road) is laid out in carpet tiles, to make it recognizable. If a child is unable to manage this bit, he is allowed to crawl...but not walk!

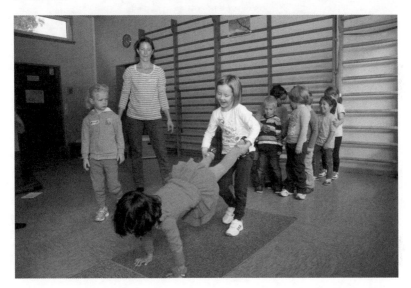

School—Fire

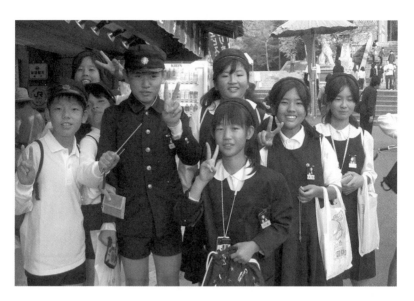

Fire Element Exercise: A popular playground game in Japan is "peg snatching." Each child is given four or five wooden clothes pins and fixes them on to their own clothing.

The task is to steal pegs from the other children and fasten them on to oneself. The game ends as soon there are children with no pegs.

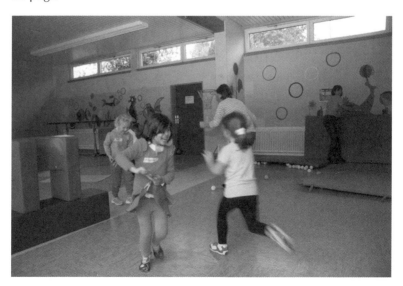

Now All the Children are Hungry for Sushi—Earth

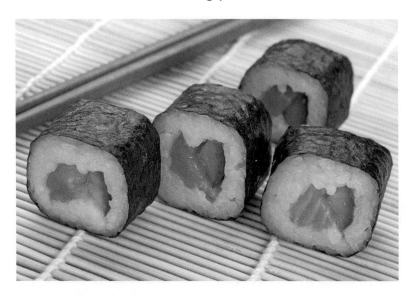

Earth Element Stimulation: The children are asked who knows what sushi is. Then sushi is explained: "It's fish with rice, wrapped up in a roll."

Earth Exercise—The Greedy Monster: The children assemble in a circle. In the middle, an imaginary table is constructed, with sushi on it. After the long journey and playtime, the children are very hungry. The children put sushi in their mouths and then stroke their hands over their mouths and faces, down the front of their bodies to the top of their feet (following the Stomach meridian), and back to their tummies. They rub their tummies—mmmmm! Repeat several times.

The Geisha Runs Along a Bench—Earth

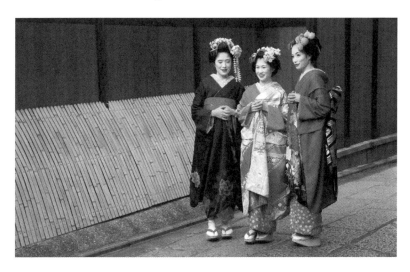

Earth Element Exercise: Each child is given a beanbag. The children place the beanbag on their heads, and hold their hands, palms together, in front of their chests. Pretending to be wearing a kimono as in the picture above, the children have to take small steps running along the bench because the kimono is very tight. If their beanbag falls off, they have to start again from the beginning. The teachers could also have the children try this backwards.

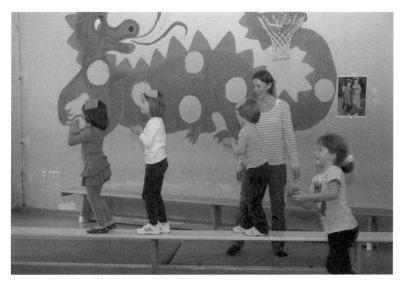

Geisha, Samurai, Dragon

Metal Element Exercise: All the children stand in a circle. Together, they practice the movements for geisha, samurai, and dragon:

- The geisha puts her hands together in front of her chest and bows.

- The samurai lunges, jerks his sword, and utters a battle cry.

- The dragon places his hands by the sides of his head and spits fire, hissing.

One child goes into the middle of the circle and says which one of the figures all the children are to imitate; then another child takes his place.

Variation: One child stands in the middle. She goes up to another child and challenges him to imitate any figure or movement that she makes—if the second child makes a mistake, he has to go into the middle.

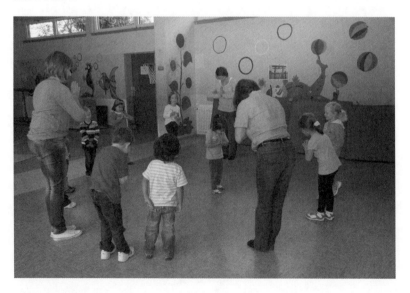

Flying Home

Water Element Exercise: All the children lie down on their backs on the mats. The plastic painter's drop cloth is wafted over the children, making the sound of air and water. The children can close their eyes if they want to and listen to the sound, or balloons can be placed in the sheets above them to watch as they move in the cloth.

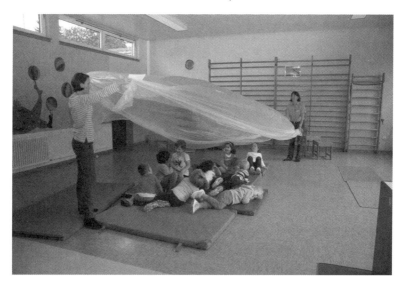

Completion

All the children sit in a circle and the following is said to them:

> You've been very courageous to make such a long journey, and you've experienced a lot along the way. We all had to think about how we were going to cross the water and then cross the mountain. At school, you were able to try out a Japanese playground game—you must have got quite warm doing that. Afterwards you all got very hungry. How did you like the sushi? Balancing with the beanbags was next—that went well. In the game with the geisha, the samurai, and the dragon, no one was hurt or devoured, because respect counts for a great deal in Japan, and even the dragon had respect.
>
> What did you like best about the journey? Think about it and then share with each other in the circle.

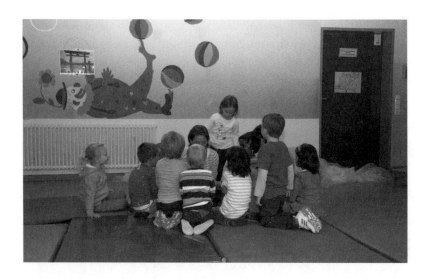

Example 4: New Sibling Adjustment—
Environmental Support and the Five Elements

This next example is about the family dynamics with a three-and-a-half-year-old named Clara, who started to wet her bed three to five times a night, sleep-walk without being able to be awakened, and had a new five-month-old brother in the home. The mother had tried monitoring how much Clara was drinking before going to bed and made sure she used the toilet; she also took Clara to the doctor to make sure no infections were present, and talked to the preschool to see if there were any new disturbances. Everything in Clara's environment was normal except for one thing: she had a new sibling, now five months old.

Discussions about the situation with a Five Element therapist revealed that Clara was very sensitive to sound and that, when the little brother cried in the car, she got very frustrated and angry at him, telling him to "shut up." The mother would very gently explain to Clara that her little brother couldn't help but cry because he didn't like to ride in the car seat and he had no other way of showing it. Clara would huff in the back seat and cross her arms, looking out the window, or cover her ears at times and scream. This made the mother even more nervous as she was driving and Clara was instructed to sit and read a book or color until they got home. Yelling/loud voice and anger are both Wood Element expressions.

Other behaviors of Clara revealed that she showed signs of needing a lot of Wood Element activities in her life; even though she was still in the *Keiraku* stage of development. She needed to draw daily, have lots of imaginary play activities, and at school enjoyed leading and creating groups of play activities with children's movie scenes. She was very decisive in what she wanted to wear, what colors she wanted in her room, and what she wanted to do during the day. The teacher reported that her sensitivity to sound often caused her to leave group activities and sit by herself to read or draw. Drawing calmed her and centered her. If the group got loud, she often put her hands over her ears.

The Five Element therapist asked how Clara was allowed to express her anger or frustration at home. The mother reported that, with all of the outlets she had to keep herself happy artistically, Clara really didn't get angry, and that the main thing that made her angry was when her little brother cried in the car. Here, the mother revealed that she didn't let Clara express her anger at her little brother, afraid she would hurt his feelings; she didn't want him to grow up thinking Clara didn't like him. The therapist asked the mother if she would be willing to let Clara yell at her brother and get angry more often in the house. She explained that the frequency of the bed-wetting was a sign of pent-up emotions that Clara really had no understanding of because she was in the *Keiraku* stage of development. She could not control what was moving inside her and at night when she was sleeping and could not control the pent up energy that was building up inside her. The mother agreed, and the next time they got in the car the mother said to Clara, "I know how angry it makes you when your little brother cries, and it's OK. If you want to yell at him today, it is all right—go ahead and do this." The mother later reported that Clara had not only yelled but she had screamed at her little brother, kicked the back of the seat, and then started to cry. All of the behaviors of anger, aggression, and tears are Wood Element expressions. The mother also reported that the little brother was so shocked at the new behavior that he laughed, which unfortunately made Clara cry harder, but it gave her more of an outlet to let her feelings out and the little brother was not harmed. Clara didn't wet her bed for the first time in weeks that first night, and as the month progressed the mother reported that, when she did occasionally wet the bed, she could locate an incident when Clara was not allowed to express her anger fully during the day before. The mother also set up other activities for Clara to release frustration in the home: pillow hitting, scribbling with a black crayon on paper and then tearing it up and throwing it away, a punching toy, and encouragement to express what was bothering her. The mother reported that Clara was not as easy a child as before, but she recognized that the bed-wetting stopped and Clara was happier and less tense overall. This is an example of looking at how the environment can block children's emotional expressions and how Five Element awareness can support simple adjustments to help a child grow.

Example 5: An Afternoon Project at Home—Five Friends

This example shows how the innate creative energy of the Five Elements can show up in the play of children and become an effortless balancing exercise as the children follow the natural cycle of the Five Elements. This session was done in the framework of an afternoon and offers creative possibilities for offering the Five Elements with different ages and in different types of settings.

The Spider's Web

Five girls, aged six to eight, and the project leader sat in an empty room in a circle around a tangled heap of different-colored yarn balls. The leader asked the girls: "What can we do with these?" An idea came quickly from one of the girls to stretch the yarn across the room. They all agreed and each child took a big handful of the yarn. Any place they could imagine could be used to attach the yarn.

The girls came up with a plan—and so they found themselves in the atmosphere of the Wood Element.

The girls busily strung the yarn from one side of the room to the other. Quickly it became hard to cross the room and the girls had to start maneuvering around the yarn by climbing over it, sliding under it, and even tossing their bundles up over the beams of the room to find room for them. When they had finished, they stepped back and admired their work from many different angles and perspectives. They climbed the wall bars to get a bird's eye view, crouched down to look through, and laid on their backs to look up and through the maze of yarn. They began to come up with new, creative ideas and the following insight presented itself: "If bells were hung from the yarn, who could move through the yarn without ringing any of the bells?"

Playfully, the children tested their sense of orientation and their physical agility, thus stimulating their Wood Element qualities.

Next, they tried gleefully to shake as many strands as possible at one time and a new idea for a game quickly unfolded: "The Spider and the Flies." The spider would stand in one corner of the room and the flies would get themselves caught and tangled in the spider's web.

When everyone was ready, the spider would start moving. As quickly as possible, the flies would have to untangle themselves and escape from the spider, while the spider tried to catch the flies. The decision was made that the girls could move only by squirming or crawling on their stomachs. After a few gleeful and screaming rounds of this, the spiders and flies alike were all hot and sweaty in the web.

They were experiencing the liveliness and exhilaration of the Fire Element.

While still sweating and catching their breath, the leader brought out a big pile of shiny strips of silk/satin cloths (these can be made from remnants from a fabric store) and a box of clothes pins. Together they thought about what to do with them. They decided to build "houses." Each girl received a pile of cloth strips of a particular color. There was a red, yellow, green, orange, and blue house. They all made sure there was enough distance between neighbors—lots of care went into making the walls. After the individual houses were ready, they all met in the middle, at the Town Square, for refreshments of cookies and cocoa.

By building the houses, the children created their place in the world, from which they could meet at a common point. This was the Earth Element expressing itself.

After their snack, they decided that it was time to go back to their own houses. Once more, they set their walls in order and some were even newly draped. They each sat in their house and could see the others inside their "walls." After a little while, the desire for contact with one another grew, and they wondered how this could be achieved. One of the girls had the idea of choosing a messenger, who was given a tube to use as a "speaking tube." Thus equipped, she went from house to house, to deliver messages. The speaker held one end to her mouth, while the listener held the other end to her ear. Whoever wished to send a message called for the messenger, gave the message, and, of course, said for whom it was intended. Again and again, the messenger had invitations to deliver messages and visit the other houses.

The houses' "walls" marked off individual boundaries and allowed the girls to sense the self-created boundaries of themselves and each other. From this experience of each other's boundaries arose the wish to meet and speak to each other. The children naturally evolved a fluid interplay between closeness and distance. They found themselves in the Metal Element expression.

During this constant visiting, the idea came to build a "townhouse" in which they could all live together. The walls of the individual houses were used to build a larger tent roof. Beneath the roof of this shared townhouse, the children made themselves comfortable. They made a resting place and snuggled together. The leader suggested that she read them a story and they all readily accepted. The afternoon together came to a close.

The children experienced their wish for closeness and quiet in the Water Element.

This Spider Web activity is an example of how children will naturally move through the Five Elements with a little guidance and support. The group leader was able to facilitate the full expression of some of the Elements—for example, cookies and cocoa, reading a book—but the children had already come to each Element on their own prior to the suggestions of the group leader.

Other Suggestions with the Spider Web Activity

A similar spider's web can be adapted to large groups outdoors or to children's birthday parties with very little space. There is no limit to the imaginative ways this can be used. A simplified form works well for parents' nights, seminars, or to loosen up other conversation circles. Participants can sit in chairs in a circle or, even better, in a circle on the floor. The following is an example of how we have used it as a ritual for getting acquainted during a parents' night. This group involved parents whose children had just started the Room to Play group in Germany and were having their first meeting out of the six they would attend while their children were active in the group.

This Spider's Web exercise was introduced for the purpose of opening conversation and getting acquainted. By going through the cycle of the Five Elements, a feeling of mutual trust and openness can be quickly established, and everyone can feel involved. One participant holds a bundle of yarn and introduces himself by name, with a short personal statement. Holding one end of the yarn, he then throws the bundle to another participant. Now this person states her name and something about herself, and holds the yarn in one hand also and passes the bundle on. The bundle of yarn keeps traveling until everyone has been introduced. Everyone is now connected to each other through the crazy maze of yarn. The group is opened.

Now it is time for questions. The leader asks the first question and throws the bundle of yarn to a participant, who answers the question and then tosses the bundle to another. Each person in turn answers the leader's question until all have replied. In the next round, a second question is asked.

Each question is designed so that it represents one of the Five Elements. Here is a sample sequence of questions:

- What helps your child most to get to sleep? (Water)

- What physical activities does your child most enjoy? (Wood)

- What do you and your child do that makes you laugh the most together? (Fire)

- In what activities do you feel closest to your child? (Earth)

- What do you respect the most about your child? (Metal)

After the last question has been answered by all participants, there is a beautiful and thickly woven web that is held by all in the group. With the yarn in hand, the participants stand up and look at the stretched web. Now, when alternate participants in the circle raise the part of the web they are holding, a fascinating three-dimensional form appears. And when every other partner passes the bundle of strands to his neighbor (so that they hold bundles in both hands— one low, one high), the "free partner" can move about in this close-meshed work of art. This demands dexterity and sometimes comical, awkward, or acrobatic movements which invariably lead to laughter. Participants can switch, so that those who held the strands now become the focus of the laughter.

By way of closing, the participants return to their places in the circle. Each now holds his/her strands. Whatever remains of the bundle of yarn is thrown back in reverse order and the maze grows—whoever wishes to can say something in turn. When the yarn bundle is completely unwound, you can fasten the web to the floor with adhesive tape and thus "preserve" the work of art for a period of time. This is especially nice in seminars lasting several days, so that one can begin and conclude with this ritual.

Ages 8–10

Example 1: A Day at the Circus

This is an example of a Spiel-Räume (Room to Play children's play therapy group) session, created by Gabriele Trinkle, practitioner of Shiatsu for babies and children.

It was completed in a session at the children's clinic with four children who had moderate attention difficulties and ranged from ages eight to ten years old. The theme of the session for the day was "A Day at the Circus."

The objective was to guide the children through all the Elements, to support the flow of any stagnant *Ki* in the Five Elements that was contributing to their difficulties. The children had not previously experienced this kind of group and this was the first of six sessions.

Materials Needed

- more balloons than there are children (ideally twice as many)

- permanent markers

- enough mats for each child to have one to lie on

- a bench or rectangular wooden blocks (about 4–6 inches wide)

- semicircular wooden blocks

- a few wobble cushions (if available—these are air-filled cushions that are not flat)

- one jump rope, or a long piece of rope

- one blanket per child

Introduction

Each member of the group blows up a balloon, fastens it with a knot, and writes their name on the balloon with a permanent marker. The balloons are tossed up in the air and away. Then each child catches a balloon, and takes it to the one whose name is written on it (since the children are new, they have to ask out loud in order to find who the balloon belongs to). Repeat this two or three times, and then set the balloons aside.

To begin the exercise, the children are asked if they have ever been to the circus and they are invited to engage in some questions for sharing: "Who's been to the circus? What did you see there? Did you like it?"

"Today in our session, you are going to be the circus performers! Let the circus begin!"

Wood Element

Familiarize the children with the materials and tell them to construct a "circus ring" in the middle of the room with the mats, semicircular and rectangular wooden blocks, perhaps a bench, and some wobble cushions for a boundary, if available. Allow the children to interact and step in and out of leading and following each other in the process.

The teacher or supervisor places a jump rope on the mats.

Transition to the Fire Element

Two supervisors (or one supervisor and a child) pick up and turn the jump rope. The children are instructed to jump through it in pairs.

Allow the children to have fun with this and pick their own partners. Next, the children take turns to fetch a balloon for each other and wait for the others to jump through the rope to start the next station.

Fire Element

Now the children are clowns during the intermissions and breaks in the circus. They move with their balloons through the circus, but are not allowed to hold them in their hands; they have to keep them moving in the air, while trying to catch the balloons of their partners! Next they "chase" the balloons while keeping them in the air in front of them, pretending they can't catch them and that the balloons keep getting away. To enliven the game, the supervisor joins in.

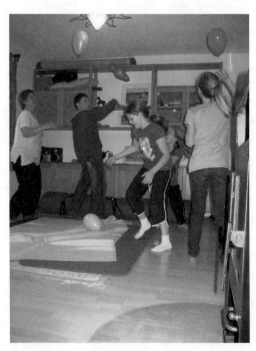

Transition to the Earth Element

The children catch their balloon and must come to a standstill with whichever balloon they have got, and try to balance it on the tip of a finger.

Earth Element

Now the children become "tightrope artists." Balancing along the rope (which the supervisor has laid out on the floor—the "tightrope"), or the wooden blocks and bench or wobble cushions, they try to balance their balloons on their fingertips.

To finish this Element, anyone who is able to can do a somersault on the soft mats in the middle of the room.

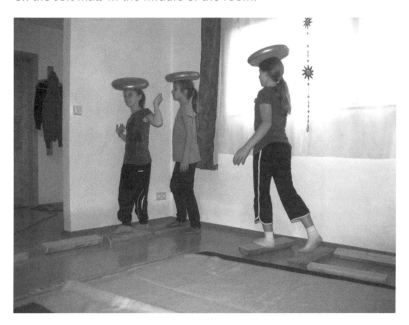

Transition to the Metal Element

The children choose a partner and take their place in the circus ring.

Metal Element

As a reward for all their strenuous activity, the artists and performers now get a balloon massage. Here the great challenge is to use the balloon in such a way that it doesn't make a squeaking noise. At the same time, they must pay attention to what their partner likes. Where would they like to be touched, and where not? How much pressure does their partner like, and for how long? Do they prefer quickly or slowly, or rolling, rubbing, or patting?

Transition to the Water Element

Each child finds a spot on a mat to lie down comfortably. They may like to be covered up, or have a blanket under their head.

Water Element

The supervisor does a fantasy dream journey with the children on the theme "A Day at the Circus." All of the Five Elements are worked with in the visualization to complete the day.

> Make yourself comfortable on the mat. Notice whether there's still something about your position that is uncomfortable that you'd like to change and then change it.
>
> Are you warm enough, or do you need a blanket?
>
> Close your eyes.
>
> Visualize yourself lying in a green meadow. The ground underneath you is pleasantly soft, and the earth is gently warmed by the spring sunshine. Here you can relax after the day's experiences. Notice your breathing—is it shallow and rapid, or slow and deep? Breathe consciously into your belly. Can you feel your ribs rising and falling?
>
> You can feel the weight of your body supported by the ground holding you up, your chest widening as you breathe in and sinking as you breathe out—rising and falling...
>
> You can feel the grass under your hands—maybe it tickles a bit. Let your hands and arms lie loose in the warm grass. Your head is lying heavy in the soft grass. The back of your neck is relaxing and getting really light. Your back is lying relaxed and heavy on the ground. Your pelvis is becoming really heavy and warm. You can feel your thighs and calves getting really relaxed, recovering from today's activity. Your heels, too, are lying really heavy on the ground.
>
> As you lie relaxing in the warm grass, images of today pass once more before you.
>
> You've been at the circus with your friends. You've had lots of fun, and a great day.

Summaries for the Children

The children are told a summary of what they did today while they lie relaxing on their mats.

WOOD

First, you helped the circus folk set up the ring. Together with your friends, you built a course for the artists and performers. On this course, you were able to try out lots of tricks for yourself. Perhaps you balanced on the tightrope—and you must have needed lots of courage and skill for that! You ran along a balance beam and practiced somersaults with the clowns. With the group of artists, you were able to try out little tricks with the skipping rope.

FIRE

At break time you and your friends played with the clowns. You chased one another's bright balloons and had lots of fun and exercise.

EARTH

You balanced balloons on your finger. That certainly wasn't easy! You got huge applause for balancing a balloon at the same time as balancing along the tightrope and the balance beam. For that trick you had to concentrate hard, so as not to lose your balloon.

METAL

As a reward for the effort, you received a balloon massage. You could feel the sensation of the balloon on your body. In some places you enjoyed it less, and in some places more. The balloons were rolled, and it was very gentle.

WATER

And at the end of the session, here you are, lying really comfortably, relaxing after all the effort and hard work. In a

while, I shall be quiet—then you can enjoy the moment's quiet.
Try to hear whether it's really completely silent.

The day at the circus is over and now it's time to go home.
You've relaxed for a bit, and are coming back slowly to the
present. You can take a good stretch... Breathe in deeply—
maybe you feel like having a loud yawn. Open your eyes, and
slowly move away from your place in the meadow. Until next
time at the circus!

Completion

Once the children are back in the "here and now," they can share
their experiences. Would they like to come to this circus again?
What would they like to experience next time?

Ages 11–14

Example 1: The Five Elements in Physical
Education—A Middle School Class (Ages 12–13)

We conducted the following project in a seventh grade middle
school class with 21 students aged 12 and 13 years. Two physical
education periods were set aside for it weekly over a period of six
months. The following goals were pursued in this project:

- Improvement of the ability to concentrate.

- Learning to listen to each other.

- Having more respect and awareness when dealing with each
  other. This focus was used because there was a situation in
  the school where aggressive behavior was occurring between
  some of the boys, and the girls were taking on the roles of
  arbitrator and mediator.

- Searching for other strategies to resolve aggressive
  confrontations.

- Improvement of physical posture and movement patterns.

The following session is an example of one of the sessions held
during the week. The following materials were needed:

- one large, empty room

- one pezzi ball (exercise ball, 24–28 inches in diameter) for each student

- three gym balls

- one large elastic cloth

- blindfolds.

Introduction Phase for the Session
The group stands in a circle. The students tap a massage on the back of the person in front of them, and then turn in the circle so that they can tap the back of the person standing behind them.

Exercises
WOOD
There is a pezzi ball for each student in the room. Each child is allowed to take one and move through the room as they wish. The question is asked: "What can we do with these?" Activities for big movements are encouraged. The group is instructed to try to crawl across the room with the ball under their belly; when someone runs into a ball or a person, they can crawl under or over.

Next, everyone takes a pezzi ball and lies on it in a prone position (on their belly), and then tries to lift their hands and feet from the ground, either alternating or all together. Those who feel confident enough can after a while attempt to turn over on to their backs without using their hands, and then return to the prone position.

FIRE
The children sit on the pezzi balls in a circle and link arms, and then roll together as far backwards and forwards as they can without breaking contact.

Then everyone drops their arms, and lies on their stomach on the ball, heads facing into the center of the circle. First one extra gym ball is rolled into the circle, then another (up to a maximum of five balls), and the group now plays "rollball," without touching their hands to the ground and making sure that the gym balls do not leave the circle as they are rolled back and forth.

EARTH

Everyone finds a comfortable spot in the room to sit on their pezzi ball. Now the object is to lift their feet off the ground and sit balanced for as long as possible without touching anyone.

Next, everyone seeks out a partner. One partner sits on the ball and tries to maintain balance, while the other pushes and pulls on the ball and tries to make the partner lose balance.

METAL

The group splits into three smaller units. While one of these smaller groups leaves the room, the second group forms into a figure and stands like a "monument." The third group spreads a cloth over this "monument" and waits nearby. Now the first group, blindfolded, is led back into the room. They must feel how the "monument" under the cloth is sitting, standing, or lying, and then imitate this "monument" using the members of the second group. When they are ready, the blindfolds and cloth are removed and the "monuments" can be compared. This is a Metal Element exercise, so the children can be reminded that their touch should be respectful; if it appears that some have difficulty with this, the teacher can guide their hands to appropriate areas for feeling the shape of the "monument."

WATER

The group divides in two. Half lie comfortably on the floor on their stomachs. The others take a pezzi ball and pick a partner from those on the floor. They roll the ball gently over the partner from head to foot. Different amounts of pressure can be tried, while asking the partner which one is preferred.

Transforming Everyday Life

To round out this chapter, we would like to give a few more examples that will show you some possibilities for integrating the Five Elements into family life. This can occur with little expense, in passing, or as a celebration with much preparation at every season. Let yourself be inspired by these suggestions, and other possibilities that occur to you. Have fun "playing" with the Five Elements!

A Craft Afternoon at Home—Spontaneous Play with Bored Children

A mother provides the following description:

An autumn afternoon. Outside, it's grayer than gray, and the chill, damp wind cuts right through every layer of clothing. The children are back from kindergarten and school, and don't feel like playing outside in this weather. Lunch and homework are all finished, and for a while the children play in their rooms— sometimes noisily, sometimes quietly. Then the doorbell rings, and a playmate for each of my sons stands there. "No, we don't want to go outside, but come on in!" There's a whole group of children gathered now, and my young daughter refuses to be left out. Stubbornly, she tries to be part of the action.

An hour later, they're all played out, and we decide to have a beautiful autumn—if not outside, then inside—and decorate the windows. There's room at the big kitchen table, so we think the idea over together: "What belongs to autumn and would be nice for us to make?" The results of our look at autumn: mist, colorful leaves, bare trees, autumn fires, hedgehogs burrowing into the ground, chestnuts, dragons, wind. And then the creative ideas quickly continue: "Who's going to make what? What do I need for this? How can I make that on the window? Where should everything go?" and so on. The children are actively engaging in the Wood Element energy.

After this is settled, we begin passing out our materials at the table, and everyone is excited to get to work. Everyone has ideas and gives his neighbors help, whether they want it or not. The energy in the room is high and the children are very active (Fire). There's not enough of some things, but since this picture is being made together, everyone has to have a bit of everything. Not everyone can do everything equally well, and so things started by one child are completed with help from the others. Everyone pitches in as best they can, and even my daughter gets to cut hedgehog spines, for which her little scissors are just great (Earth).

Time goes by and the windows become brighter and brighter with the children's decorations. Those who have finished can see that what they have made is part of the whole and, at the same time, is pretty by itself (Metal). We get all bundled up and go outside to admire our work. It looks so great that it almost doesn't matter that the sky is blue only inside our house, that the clouds have thick whiskers, and the dragon is flying between colored leaves on the window. There is acceptance of what has been made by all (Metal).

All the children were worn out after this and the mother was left to clean up. The guests left for home and, in the mother's words, her little "warriors" were tired and ready for a quiet activity (Water).

Autumn Walk
Another Five Element experience was reported by a mother in the following description:

> We pulled on our thick coats and rubber boots to take an autumn walk. We went a little way into the woods and stopped to think about it for a few minutes: "What looks like autumn? How do we imagine autumn?" The children had—as usual—very concrete ideas about what they saw.
>
> Together we went looking for something that we liked about autumn. A change has come over many of the trees, leaving them with bare branches. Every time we see a bare tree standing alone, we think about what kind of pictures it reminds us of. One tree looks like a little squirrel, another like a monster, and two others are so close together it's as if they are holding hands (Wood).
>
> Yes, we agree that what we like about autumn is that it has so many changes, and everyone shares an idea of what changes they recognize as they see it (Fire). As we continued to walk, fruits were lying on the ground, and the accompanying children's wagon turned into a freight wagon, and the children's pants and coat pockets got filled, too (Earth). Autumn can be so colorful, even on the grayest day.
>
> What animals eat all this? Who relies on these fruits? And the trees—what are they doing now that they've lost their leaves? Well, even a tree must rest sometimes.

Back at home we dump our treasures on a big cloth, and there's lots more than just dirt. Everyone must pick out one piece that's especially important to them (Metal). After we have all admired each other's treasures, everyone plants an acorn, a maple seed, a beech nut, and a chestnut. We place the leaves in a thick coloring book. Then we all head inside and snuggle down on the couch, because the cool air and all that running made us tired (Water).

Season Tables

The season table is another very beautiful possibility for integrating and experiencing the Elements in everyday family life. There are numerous books with many suggestions for this in the context of Waldorf education (see the Resources section for more information). The season table gives children a chance to make a place in the house where they can witness the cycle of the seasons of the year.

Each season will prompt its own suggestions about the shaping of the season table, such as things from nature we find on walks outdoors, or little craft projects, or even a simply formed doll. The whole thing can be arranged with a root, bark, or a fully grown piece of wood on suitably colored cloths. The season table will soon become a place where the children will stop and look or think for a moment, wondering how they can remodel it so that it expresses the new changes that have taken place in nature. It is important that the season table remain in a fixed place within the home, and not be moved back and forth.

The following are some suggestions for making a season table (once you have begun, other ideas will come all by themselves).

Wood

Wood time is the time of spring, and if you look up the spring solstice in a calendar it will show the dates that the sun and earth move into spring out of winter. At first, there is not much to be seen above ground, but underneath, unseen, the seeds are stirring. Accordingly, the colors of the cloths on our season table are delicate and refined. Reflecting the outside when the first snowdrop flowers show themselves, the first delicate shoots of green can be seen coming up from the ground, often through the last snow, and the branches on the trees show little buds of life. When spring really arrives, there are many yellows and shades of green. Narcissuses, violets, tree blossoms—all still delicate and hazy. The table should reflect the colors and feelings of spring. At Easter time, of course, eggs, rabbits, and hens will be included.

Fire

Now summer comes in with strong colors—everything is in bloom. Everything is buzzing and humming, and the first fruits begin to appear. Outdoors, nature gives us magnificent bunches of flowers for the season table. Let the children add to the table what makes them think of summer.

Earth

In nature, fruits are ripening, everything is found in abundance, and yet the colors are already a bit subdued. A hint of autumn can be felt. The time for the harvest festival draws near. On the table, there are more shades of ocher, yellow, and brown. Little twigs and clumps of moss also look nice here.

Metal

The harvest has been gathered. Fruits, seeds, nuts, chestnuts, little gourds, early turning leaves, or handcrafted mushrooms now decorate the table. Rosehips and autumn flowers or perhaps a few pine cones will complete the picture. The children also like to make little paper kites that hang from the ceiling above the table. At Halloween, a small jack-o'-lantern can be added.

Water

Now all of nature has withdrawn into itself and is in its winter sleep. Beautifully or bizarrely formed twigs and branches, a root that is home to a dwarf, interesting stones, and dried leaves all express this. A deep blue cloth with hand-made snowflakes can be scattered on the table. Of course, the season table also encompasses the family traditions of Hanukkah, Christmas, or other religious rituals that the family celebrates, with golden stars, angels, a St Nicholas, nativity, or handmade ornaments—whatever the children want to add to the table to express the season.

These are just a few of many possibilities for making a season table. Children can develop a wealth of ideas for constantly renewing this family spot, particularly when they sense that everyone takes pleasure from it. Enjoy being creative and spontaneous with the Five Elements in your homes and your lives.

CHAPTER 14

Touching Community
A Five-Week Project and Community Event

This chapter offers two examples that take a little more effort and planning but can have a wonderful and rewarding effect with the number of individuals they can reach and support. Our hope is to offer more ways to be creative in the Five Elements so that you are inspired to carry this out in your community.

A Five-Week Journey through the Five Elements: A Course for Children Ages 4–5

Some of these ideas are from the final projects of students training as baby and child Shiatsu therapists, as well as teachers, in Germany. Here we would like to express our warmest thanks to our colleagues Iris Bungert and Ruth Pontius for this project.

The following course was run in the Stennweiler Children's Daycare Center within the town kindergarten of the parish of Schiffweiler. It can be adapted to an older age group by changing the theme and activities to appropriate age levels. Our experience shows us that, once the group begins, the movement of the Five Elements is contagious and people of all ages can't resist participating and enjoying something that naturally moves within them.

There are a couple of important aspects about this Five Element five-week project with four- to five-year-olds that are different and even contrary to what we shared in Chapter 10 about the guidelines for working with children and the Five Elements. First, this example was offered to children not yet in this stage of Five Element energetic development. The 4–5-year-olds who participated in this activity were in the active stages of *Keiraku* motor development as discussed in Chapter 1. We have decided to include this project so as to offer you, the reader, an opportunity to see how children can still work with the Five Elements when the leaders/adults have a good understanding of child development and are able to follow three important guidelines:

1. The leaders must understand that the children are not capable of expressing age-appropriate Five Element responses to the exercises offered. Expectations need to be lowered and the children allowed to play and experiment with the story and exercises.

2. Exercises with a lot of movement opportunities must be offered for the children to express the *Keiraku* stage of development that corresponds with the Elements. Examples are provided for this.

3. The adults/leaders must provide the environment of each Element and become the examples of the Element qualities so that the children can experience what is innate within them and begin to see new possibilities for how to express the Five Elements.

A second feature you might recognize in the following example that is different from what is written earlier in the book is that this example does not begin in the traditional order of the Five Elements. This example begins the first week with the Earth Element and then follows another ancient order of working with the Five Elements from a different Japanese tradition.

This tradition works with the theory that it is beneficial for the Earth Element to be offered at the beginning of the exercise, followed by a crossing pattern of the sequence of Elements that supports the opposite directions of their energy flow. This can help younger children who have not reached the developmental stage of the Five Elements because it uses the Earth Element characteristics which are a strong part of the Front Family characteristics.

The Front Family is the first energy pattern that infants experience when they come into their center and begin the stage of integrating their self-awareness separate from others. Therefore, when one starts in the Earth Element, it accesses the very early pattern of the energy flow in the body and offers the most developed and grounded awareness developed in an individual at that time.

For this reason, it could also be beneficial to use this elemental sequence for groups that are dealing with the themes of PTSD, grief, or other experiences that have left some shock or emotional trauma that the movement of the energy in the Five Elements could support clearing. Since the Earth Element has the theme of safety and finding one's feet on the ground, starting with this Element is an advantage for individuals struggling with normalizing after very difficult experiences in life.

There are other traditions and ways to offer the Five Element sequence, and we have chosen not to elaborate on these but to focus primarily on the order we have had the most success with over the years. Our hope in including this variation is to show that there are other very skillful ways to work with the Five Elements and that children can be supported in expanding their capacity in different ways.

The Five-Week Project

For this course, a large, empty room was used. All participants were dressed in comfortable clothes and non-slip socks or gym shoes. A mat and a blanket were laid out ready for each child.

General Structure of the Course

We chose to begin with the Earth Element in order to activate the themes of inner safety, centering, security, nourishing, and being nourished. If the Earth Element is strengthened, participants are able to find their center and feel safe in the exercises. For young children or participants who have difficulty with this aspect in their life, it can support them and help them feel safe and at home in the group.

The following diagram represents the order in which the Five Elements were offered during the five weeks:

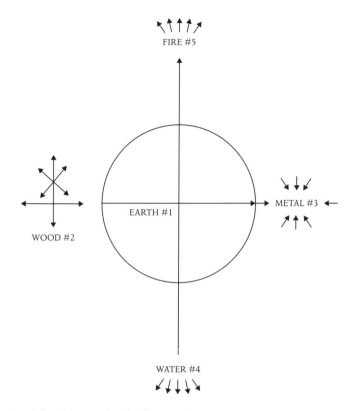

Order of the Elements for the five-week course

Preparing for the Element Sessions

The following sequence was used with each of the Element sessions.

Before the start of the session, an "island" was created in a corner of the room to represent the Element of the week, with colors and a story that gave the children a sense of the theme of the Element in their lives. The purpose of this island was to represent the Element to the children, using all the senses:

- taste—food

- smell—scents, flowers, spices

- sight—images, objects

- touch—touching the objects

- hearing—stories, noises (e.g. singing bowls).

The children's mats were laid out in a circle in the middle of the room. Inside the circle a centerpiece was arranged, corresponding with the Element being stimulated and focused on for that week. Anything that could help the children to get a feeling for the Element was used—for example, colored fabric; natural materials from the corresponding season such as wood, grass, moss, leaves, shells, stones, and feathers; our own photos; and pages from old calendars or postcards. In addition, a space was created in the room for the children to retire to in case they needed a break during the session. The following is an outline of the steps that were taken to work with the Element in each session.

The Sessions

Each session followed the same sequence and plan:

1. *Entering into the Element experience:* The leaders and the children come together on the mats to begin exploring the Element of the week.

   a. A centerpiece for the Element of the week was created by the leaders, and the children were invited to look, touch, and talk about the centerpiece. It is important to note that the focus is to allow the children to discover and describe what they see and feel.

   b. The group leader briefly introduces the Element for the week on a level that is appropriate for the age level of the students by navigating the exploration of the children to arrive at the Element being worked with.

2. A power animal or character relating to the Element is presented that will work with the theme for the rest of the session. The children are invited to change into the power animal/character with a description of what they are like from the leaders.

3. The leaders describe a fantasy island where the children will be going—a land to experience the Element of that week.

4. A "tuning-in" exercise to awaken the Element in each child is done with the group interacting with one another as their power/character animal. Movement is involved here.

5. A story is read out loud to the children that relates to the Element and the power animal.

6. The experimental phase consists of exercises to stimulate and strengthen the Element of the week and the corresponding meridians. The exercises are chosen and introduced in a way that is appropriate to the story.

7. The children visit and discover the land of the Element for that week with various foods and objects to give the senses the experience of the Element.

8. If the children want to experience Shiatsu (Japanese acupuncture massage) during the session, it is offered at this point. The meridians that correspond to the Element of the week are worked on with the children. Either two children treat each other or all the children lie down and receive treatment from the course leaders who are licensed bodywork therapists. No matter which way Shiatsu is offered, before the children are touched, they are always asked whether they would like to be touched. Children could also be shown how to work on the meridian pathways themselves (e.g. using a tennis ball to roll up and down the meridians).

Note: Shiatsu massage is typically done on a mat on the floor through clothing. The touch with Shiatsu comes from applying relaxed pressure with your own bodyweight on to the receiver. When learning how to use this kind of touch, it's necessary to learn and practice first in the all-fours position. The children crawl around the room, learning and practicing how to distribute their weight evenly on their hands and knees. This also applies when "treating" a partner—for example, in moving the palm of a hand along a leg or arm or the back of the child being treated, your weight is distributed evenly on all four weight-bearing points (both knees and both hands) at once. In the course that is described in this example, the course leaders treated the children with Shiatsu. Other tools can be used so that the children can treat themselves.

9. Change the children back into children as they come out of their power animal.

10. The closing ritual is completed for the Element that week.

- To give the children the opportunity to remember and express the Elements at home as well as in the classroom, a set of small cards were made for this course. The power animal for the Element goes on the front of the cards, and on the reverse side are the three empowering sentences that were created for that Element. In addition, after the session, each child receives a "symbol" of the Element for that session.

- All the symbols, together with the empowerment cards, make up the contents of a little "treasure chest" that each child receives.

The Journey Through the Five Elements
FIRST WEEK: THE EARTH ELEMENT—"THE SHIRE"

1. *Entering into the Earth Element experience:*

   a. The leaders and the students all sit together in a circle around the centerpiece created by the leaders for the Earth Element, and the children look at, touch, and talk about what they can see in the images.

   The centerpiece is composed of the following: yellow and orange fabrics; a pumpkin; a sunflower; a small sponge cake or cookie; and postcards, your own photographs or or pages from an old calendar showing friendly faces, lush, ripe fields, or people bringing in the harvest, holding hands.

   b. The leaders add to the discussion of what the children are expressing and discovering about the Element in the centerpiece, keeping the meaning of the Element in mind while giving free rein to the imagination and not forgetting that the children need to have the meaning explained to them. Their images, sensations, and questions were related to the Earth Element to offer a more rounded picture of what the Earth Element is.

2. *The fantasy land of the Earth Element — describing the Shire:*

    The Shire appears as a fair and gentle landscape with rolling hills. There are fields of ripe, golden corn, and green meadows where cows, goats, and sheep are grazing. In the orchards and fruit fields are ripe, juicy fruits waiting to be harvested, like grapes, peaches, oranges, and apples. The inhabitants of the Shire are dwarves—they live in comfy caves and it is very important to them that they get to eat nice, tasty meals each day. They love their snug homes, and they don't like adventures at all.

3. *Transformation into the Earth power animal/character — bears:*

    In order to get to the Shire safely, we are going to change ourselves into nice, sweet bears for the journey. Now each of you as a bear snuggles into your cave. We bears like having our fur stroked and this makes us feel good in our bodies. We make a big, comfortable yawn and a good stretch.

4. *Tuning-in exercise for the Earth Element:*

    Now all the bears are leaving their caves to go and meet the other bears. In a little glade in the forest all the bears meet up and greet one another happily. All together, they start singing a song: "The Bare Necessities" (from *The Jungle Book*). After a round of the song in the circle, all the bears go back to their places to listen to the story.

5. *Story reading for the Earth Element:*

    Growling happily, with a song on their lips, the bears set off for the Shire. It's a fine afternoon. The bees are buzzing in the air, the sun is shining warm on the bears' noses, and the leaves they eat along the way are fresh and really warm in their mouths. The bears trot along through the peaceful forest and gather sweet, juicy forest fruits as a gift for the dwarves.

But soon, from far off, dark clouds approach. They sense that soon there's going to be a storm. Rather worried, they wonder whether they will make it to the Shire before the storm breaks—the first raindrops are falling already. Quickly, they trot onwards and arrive in the Shire dripping wet, before the storm really breaks out in loud thunder and lightning.

The bears get a warm welcome from the dwarves and find shelter from the storm in the cozy caves. Concerned about the bears' health, the dwarves hurry away to fetch fluffy towels and warm blankets. They dry the bears' dripping fur and serve them hot tea and sweet-smelling honey cake. For dessert, they eat the sweet berries they picked in the forest.

After such a delicious meal, everyone is content and happy, and they sit together for a long time. When the bears leave, the dwarves give each of them a little pot of the delicious honey as a memento of their lovely afternoon together.

6. *The experimental phase—exercises to strengthen the Earth Element:*

   a. *Bear and cave.* The children form pairs. One child is the bear and kneels on the floor, while the other child stands behind him and stretches out his arms over his partner, to make a cave for the bear. The bear gets a sense of how much shelter he needs. The child pretending to be the cave adapts to the bear's needs, sensing how much shelter the bear needs. Here, the theme of the Earth Element being expressed is that of caring and being cared for.

   b. *Circling the hips.* The children all loosen their hips by rotating their hips in circles. This releases tension and allows them to sense the center of the body.

   c. *Mountain pose.* The children stand upright with their legs at hip-width apart. The pelvis is centered (check that they don't have a hollow back!); they keep their shoulders back and slightly down, allowing the chest to open in front; the arms hang loose at the sides; and the head is relaxed in the center, with the neck appearing to stretch up without effort from the lengthening spine. This exercise should give the children a sense of balance and stability (standing like a mountain). Once the children have a sense of their center, the course leader (with the children's permission) gently and playfully nudges them off balance.

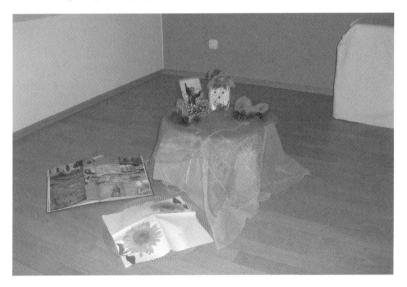

7. *Discovering the Earth Element land.* The following items and foods are set up for the children to taste, touch, smell, and examine the Earth Element with their senses: yellow and orange color scheme; honey, a carrot, and a banana; vanilla scent; and tree bark, moss, and fir cones.

8. *Shiatsu.* The children are asked: "Which of you bears would like to have your fur stroked?" Those bears then lie down on their backs on their mats. The course leader crawls on all fours up to the first child and places beanbags along the front of their legs and body (along the Stomach and Spleen meridians), but not on the face. Then the leader "crawls" with her hands over the beanbags. It is important for the leader

(or the student if the children are working on each other) to pay attention to make sure the pressure is coming from their relaxed bodyweight as they do this. Each child wanting the Shiatsu receives the treatment. If touch is not allowed between teacher and students, the children can be shown how to stimulate the meridians with a tennis ball and then lie down with a heavy blanket, pillows, or beanbags resting on the stomach meridian.

9. *Changing back into children.* The little bears cover themselves up with a blanket if not already covered. The course leader crawls to each child in turn, strokes the blanket, or the air above it, lightly and says: "Now the brown bear (polar bear, teddy bear, koala bear) is turned back into girl XX [child's name] or boy XY from the Frog Group [name of the kindergarten group]." The children are asked to remain lying down until all the bears have been changed back into children.

10. *Closing ritual.* The children form a circle. As a memento of the session they receive a little pot of honey for their treasure chests and a card with a picture of a bear on the front side and the three empowerment statements on the back. All together they say the following empowerment sentences three times:

- I am full.

- I feel safe.

- I enjoy helping others.

SECOND WEEK: DESCRIBING THE WOOD ELEMENT— THE JUNGLE, LAND OF ADVENTURE

1. *Entering into the Wood Element:*

   a. Everyone sits together in a circle around the centerpiece created for the Wood Element and the children look and say what they recognize in the images. The centerpiece is composed of the following: fabrics in shades of green; a piece of tree bark; a paint box and paintbrushes; postcards, your own photos, or pictures from old calendars showing a weightlifter; pictures of a galloping horse or eyes (of animals or people); image of a cave; and pictures of a meadow in spring or a hissing tiger.

b. The leaders support the exploration, keeping the meaning of the Wood Element in mind while giving free rein to the children's imagination and not forgetting that the children need to have the meaning explained to them. The group gives presence to the Wood Element and gains access to the particular "place" that needs to be explored during the session.

2. *Transformation into the Wood Element power animal— tiger children.* To begin, the children set up a den with their blankets and lie down on them. The course leaders crawl to each child in turn and touch them (ask first!), saying: "Lucy, [insert child's name] or girl (or boy) in the Frog Group [name of the kindergarten group] now becomes a little tiger that's still fast asleep."

3. *Describing the Wood island—the jungle.* As the children lie on their blankets, the jungle is described in the following words: "Early in the morning the jungle awakes. The parrots and cockatoos start squawking; the elephants greet the day with their trumpeting trunks. Butterflies of every color fly through the air, and the wind blows through the luminous green canopy of the giant, ancient trees. The tiger children wake up too, and feel the wind blowing gently through their silky-soft fur."

4. *Tuning-in exercise for the Wood Element.* The "cat stretch" is used to extend and stretch their muscles and sinews and the tiger children roll and stretch in their den. The tigers are told to show their claws. The tiger children prowl about the jungle (the room) and show their claws to the other children when they meet. Softly with the palms of their hands, the children strike the inside of the legs at the ankles and drag them up the

legs to an upright position, where they then gnash their teeth and claw at the air with their hands.

5. *Story reading.* The children return to their mats to listen to the story:

> Early in the morning, with the wind blowing through their fur, the tiger children wake up. They roll and stretch and, in one bound, leap up out of their den. They are really excited, because today they are to go deep into the jungle, to the mysterious waterfall. They have heard that anyone who bathes in this waterfall grows very strong and brave and can roar like a big, powerful tiger.
>
> Softly, without waking their mother, they set off. Suddenly there's a deafening noise and, really scared, they hide behind a big tree. And look! Bamboo, the elephant, comes out of the thicket, flapping his big ears. On his trunk sits a gorgeous green butterfly, beating its wings in preparation for take-off. Really relieved, the tiger children come out of hiding, for Bamboo is their friend. They play together for a bit, before setting off once more on their way to the waterfall. They get tired and lie down for a rest.
>
> Then they hear a low but clear hissing sound— zzzzssss, zzzzssss, zzzzssss. A green python slithers up, on the look-out for a tasty breakfast. Anxiously, the little tigers duck into the long grass until the python has gone. Phew! That worked!
>
> Now the tiger children hurry to get to the waterfall, as they can already hear, in the distance, the sound of water rushing. Only a few meters further, and there they are. The waterfall is truly beautiful and glistens in every color. Delighted, the little tigers jump into the cool wetness and feel themselves getting big, strong, and brave. Now they won't need to hide from a python anymore!
>
> Soon they leave the waterfall, to get home before dark. Eagerly, they tell their mother about their adventures

in the jungle and the mysterious waterfall. They rear up tall, show their claws, and roar like powerful tigers: "Wrrraaah!!!" Their mother says: "I'm proud of you for going into the jungle all by yourselves and coming back with the courage and strength of big tigers. Now you must be hungry! Look, I've got something ready for you to eat."

6. *The experimental phase—exercises to strengthen the Wood Element:*

   a. *The triangle.* Stand upright with legs apart. Raise outstretched arms to shoulder level, with the palms of the hands facing down towards the floor. As you breathe out, bend to the right until the hand of your outstretched right arm reaches your foot (or as far as you can). Look in the direction of your left hand. On the next out-breath, straighten up again, and then repeat on the opposite side. Throughout the exercise, your two arms are in a straight line. The bottom mustn't stick out too much. (The effect of this is to stretch the Gall Bladder meridian.)

   b. *The tiger sharpens its claws.* Stand upright with legs apart. Stretch your arms up to the ceiling, with the palms of your hands facing each other. With arms outstretched, lean with your upper body first to the right and then to the left. As soon as you are standing straight again with your arms stretched at the center position, leap forward in one bound, bringing your arms in front of your body and making claws with your fingers. This is accompanied by loud hissing and gnashing of teeth.

   c. *Look-out.* The children make a telescope with their hands, and use it to search for the whereabouts of the waterfall or other animals in the jungle.

   d. *Adventure trail/obstacle course.* The children are given the idea that there is a special treasure chest in the jungle and they need to create a path to get to it. Give them a variety of things to choose from to create their own obstacle course in the jungle to get to the chest. The chest is a box or bag that they will reach into without knowing or seeing what it is inside.

Before this test of courage they are guided again through the exercise "The tiger sharpens its claws." Then each child reaches into the chest and receives a card with an optical illusion—in this case, a small tiger inside a big tiger—to educate their sense of sight. (Optical illusion pictures can be accessed on the internet; you can copy the pictures on to paper and make the cards yourself.)

7. *Exploring the Wood Element land.* The following items and foods are set up for the children to taste, touch, smell, and examine the Wood Element with their senses: green color scheme; a green apple, a lime, and a live, potted mint plant; and an optical illusion (the tiger card explained above).

8. *Shiatsu.* The children lie on their sides, and beanbags are laid along the Gall Bladder meridian. The weight of the beanbags helps the children to get a better sense of the side of their body. If the children wish, they receive Shiatsu treatment along the Gall Bladder meridian or use the tennis ball to roll down their Gall Bladder meridians.

9. *Changing back into children.* All the tigers return to their places and the course leaders change them back into children.

10. *Closing ritual.* The children form a circle. As a memento of the session, following the test of courage, they receive the optical illusion card and their power card with a picture of a tiger on one side and the empowerment statements on the other. All say each of the following sentences together three times:

- I am brave.

- I am strong.

- I know what I want.

THIRD WEEK: DESCRIBING THE METAL ELEMENT— WHITE FEATHER, BLACK STAR

1. *Entering into the Metal Element:*

    a. Everyone sits together in a circle around a Metal Element centerpiece and the children look and say what they recognize and connect with their discovery. The centerpiece is composed of the following: white fabric; a singing bowl or other metal object; a few feathers; dried autumn leaves or chestnuts; postcards or pages from old calendars showing an eagle or clear windowpanes or crystals; a picture showing a clear blue sky or an autumn landscape; and pictures conveying a sense of freedom (flying birds, someone flying a kite or standing on the summit of a mountain…).

    b. Supporting and guiding the discovery and exploration with the children, the group gives presence to the Metal Element and gains access to the particular "place" that needs to be explored during the session.

2. *Describing the Metal land—a Native American village:*

    The village of the Native American children lies in a sheltered valley, close to a river and a shady forest. It's autumn already, and the forest is glowing with its bright autumn colors in the dusk lighting. The Native American children have to go to kindergarten or school in the early evening as well, as they have a lot to learn—for example, how to read animal tracks, riding, smelling danger, approaching by stealth, and shooting with a bow and arrow.

3. *The Metal Element power character—transformation into Native American children.* The children set out their beds and lie down for a midday rest. They are changed one after the other into Native American children. For this, "warpaint" is applied to each child's face, using make-up. (Always ask first, and take care to use hypoallergenic make-up!) Another possibility is to give the child a headband made from a strip of cardboard and decorated with a bright feather.

4. *Tuning-in exercises for the Metal Element:*

   a. *Bow and arrow.* The children stand up straight, take one step forward with their left leg, and bend the knee; the back leg is stretched out behind. At the same time they fix their gaze on the target they want to hit. The left arm, holding the invisible bow, is stretched out in front. The right arm tenses the bow and is drawn towards the chest, parallel with the left arm. The children have to notice the level of physical tension in their bodies before releasing the bow and shooting the invisible arrow.

   b. *Blowing on the fire.* The children are instructed to blow a small feather for a short distance. As they do this, they have to be aware of their breathing and regulate it appropriately.

   c. *Clapping rhythm.* All kneel together in a circle. The course leaders clap a rhythm—for example, clap hands once, clap on the floor once. Once all the children can follow the rhythm, it is changed—for example, clap hands once, clap on the floor twice.

5. *Story reading:*

   After evening school, all the Native American children leap around happily and play together. Only White Feather sits sad and silent at the edge of the forest and gazes longingly at the horse paddock. There stands Black Star, the horse he so much wanted, which his father had given him the week before. But Black Star appears not to like him, for every time White Feather approaches him, he gallops away. White Feather longs to ride Black Star along the river, but Black Star runs frantically around the horse paddock, bucking and blowing air heavily out of his nose, keeping a distance and big boundary between him and White Feather every time he tries to get close.

Over and over again, no matter how often he tries, his horse runs away. What is he to do? He's really desperate! He'd like to ask his father for advice, but the grown-ups haven't got time—they're gathering fruit and nuts for the approaching winter, and the tents need repairing.

So White Feather decides to look for his friend, the eagle. The wise eagle has helped him often. The eagle lives high up in the mountain, and the next day White Feather sets off to see his friend. He goes upstream along the deep valley, past fields and tall trees that glow with the widest variety of autumn colors you can imagine. He hopes that his friend will be able to help him this time too! Now the path is narrow and full of stones, rising higher and higher. The air up here is fresh and clear—ah! It feels good.

White Feather gazes up at the sky, looking for his friend, and there he is! Majestically, he flies through the air with outspread wings. Now only a few meters further, and White Feather finally reaches the eagle's look-out perch. He waves to his friend. The eagle, who spotted him a long time ago, swoops down to land next to him.

"You're here, my friend, what brings you to me?" White Feather tells the wise eagle about the trouble he's having with his horse.

"I can understand that this makes you sad, my friend. But look, you must give your horse the time he needs to get used to you. You shouldn't storm around him. He isn't used to people, because before your father caught him, he was used to moving around the open plains, with no boundaries, wild and free. Already the paddock feels too close for his boundaries, and when you get closer he gets even wilder to get more space. You must tame him slowly, very slowly. Your horse needs you to show him you respect his boundaries and that you give him space and time to get comfortable with you and choose when he can get closer to you. Only try to get a little closer every day. Respect the distance he still needs; if he gets anxious, back away and give him space again. Walk around the paddock with the other horses, and let him feel you in the space with all of them. Have patience! You'll see that he'll start to learn to feel comfortable with you in his paddock space more and more, and one day he'll eat out of your hand. Don't give up—your horse likes you, for certain! I'm glad you've shared your trouble with me and that I was able to advise you, but now go home, your horse is waiting for you." Thankful and full of hope, White Feather takes leave of his friend.

When he gets back, White Feather follows his friend's advice and slowly, cautiously, day by day, he makes friends with his horse. And so Black Star and White Feather become close friends and go through many adventures together.

6. *The experimental phase—exercises to strengthen the Metal Element:*

    a. *Bow and arrow.* The children stand up straight and take a step forwards with their left leg; the front knee is bent; and the back leg remains straight. At the same time, they fix their gaze on the target they want to hit. Now the left arm (the arm holding the invisible bow) is stretched out in front. The right arm tenses the bow, becoming parallel with the left arm as it is pulled back towards the chest. The children should notice the tension in their bodies before releasing their bow and shooting the invisible arrow.

    b. *Greeting Great Manitou (Great Spirit).* The children stand up straight and stretch up, reaching up with their arms, and breathing in deeply as they do so. As they breathe out, they let their arms drop to the ground, go into a squat, and make themselves really small.

c. *Coming close/backing away—sensing "Safe Space."* Two children stand opposite one another. One child is the horse, the other the Native American boy. Step by step, the Native American boy slowly approaches the horse. If the horse feels that the boy is getting too close, he says "Stop!"

d. *Tracing the outline of the body with a rope.* The children go into pairs. One of them lies down on their mat. The other child uses a rope to outline the body of the one who is lying down. Then the children who are lying down get up, and all the children look at the rope outlines and try to identify which one belongs to which child. You could consider any special points with the children: body positions or humorous details such as a ponytail.

7. *Visiting and exploring the Metal Element island.* The following items and foods are set up for the children to experience the Metal Element with their senses: white color scheme; hot spices such as ginger or chili; nuts and dried fruit; frankincense and spruce essential oils; and feathers.

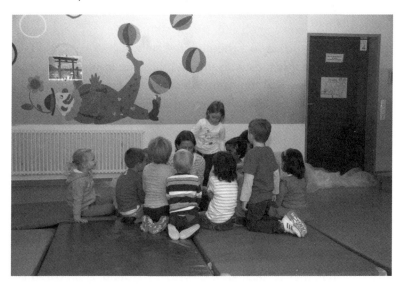

8. *Shiatsu.* The Native Americans who want to be touched lie down on their backs on their camp beds (mats). The course leaders crawl up to each child in turn and apply pressure with their hands (as previously described) along the course of the Lung and Large Intestine meridians in the arms or the children use a tennis ball to stimulate the meridian and then lie down.

9. *Changing back into children.* All the Native American children go back to their places and are tapped by the course leader to change them back into their normal selves.

10. *Closing ritual.* The children form a circle. As a memento of this session, they receive a feather for their treasure chest. All together they speak the following empowerment sentences, each three times:

- I know my limits.

- I know your limits.

- I am thankful for good friends.

FOURTH WEEK: DESCRIBING THE WATER ELEMENT—THE GREAT SEA TURTLE

1. *Entering into the Water Element:*

   a. Everyone sits in a circle around a Water Element centerpiece. The children look and say what they recognize in the images. The centerpiece is composed of the following: fabrics in shades of blue; postcards, your own photos, or pages from old calendars with an image of an old person; pictures of water in various states (icicles, snowscape, tumultuous waves, calm lake); pictures of an old turtle, a cemetery, or a newborn baby; and pictures that convey a sense of relaxation, trust, or fear.

   b. Supporting and guiding the discovery and exploration with the children, the group gives presence to the Water Element and gains access to the particular "place" that needs to be explored during the session.

2. *Describing the Water land—Island in the sea:*

    Today we are going to an island in the sea. This island has a wide, sandy beach, and beyond it a coastline of massive cliffs. In the rocks there are large and small caves where cranes have built their nests. In the water around and on the island there is a deep, silent, underwater world—here the water shimmers in countless shades of blue.

3. *Transformation into Water Element power animals—great, wise sea turtles.* All the children lie curled up under their blankets on their mats. "You are lying buried deep in the sand, for during a cold, starlit night your mother has laid you as turtle eggs in this nest of sand. Inside your egg you are aware of the silence, and of being alone. You're a bit scared of something unknown and begin consciously breathing in and out. You grow calm and your fear vanishes. As time goes on you feel cramped inside your egg and want to get out of the shell." The children begin to move and stretch out their arms and legs, getting a sense of their bodies. "Once you've hatched, you struggle upwards through the sand." The children sit down on their blankets.

4. *Tuning-in exercise for the Water Element.* To activate their energy, the children rock to and fro on their backs. They wrap their arms around their legs, which are bent at the knees. Then they hold on to their left foot with their right hand, and their right foot with their left hand, and rock to and fro on their backs again.

    After this the children sit upright with their legs outstretched, and stretch their arms upwards. Finally, they bend over with their arms stretched out to touch their toes. Here, someone could be like a stone tumbling in the river or waterfall, feeling the way the power of the water shapes and moves them.

5. *Story reading:*

    In the distance, the little turtle can hear the rushing of the sea. It would like to get there, into the safety of the water. It doesn't yet know how it will manage to tackle the long distance across the beach to the sea, all on its own. But deep inside, it feels able to trust. Everything should turn out well in good time.

The night is clear, starry, and cold as the little turtle sets off on its way to the sea. It's a bit afraid of what might happen on the way—a crane might spot it, or a snake or a crocodile—and each time it thinks about that, it moans softly to itself.

Suddenly, close to the little turtle, something moves, and its limbs twitch with fright. It can tell by the hissing sound that a snake is approaching. The little turtle starts to quiver. It's afraid that it won't be fast enough to get away from the snake. However, fear is also the little turtle's strength, and so, very carefully, it retreats inside its shell and sits as still as a stone in the sand. The snake doesn't recognize it and slithers noiselessly past.

The little turtle is out of danger. The snake must have picked up the scent of something else to eat. The turtle supposes that life is always like this, and always will be. Every creature has to survive, and has to take care not to be eaten by another.

The little turtle continues on its way to the sea, and after a while the sand grows firmer under its feet. Here comes a big, gentle wave rolling up the shore, and carries it into the sea. The tension of the little turtle's dangerous journey drops away, and it dives, relaxed and joyful, to meet its brothers and sisters and hear what they have to tell about their journeys.

6. *The experimental phase—exercises to strengthen the Water Element:*

   a. *Turtle and rattlesnake.* The children get into pairs. One child is the turtle and crouches on their mat with their back to the other child. Their partner is the rattlesnake and kneels in front of the child who is crouching. Holding a rattle in her hand, she starts to shake it along the back of the crouching child, without touching her. On hearing the rattle, the crouching child stiffens—once the rattle is silent, the crouching child can relax again. Then the turtle child consciously looks to see who the rattlesnake is.

b. *Greeting/dance of the little turtles.* Two children stand opposite one another and hold hands. They kneel down both at once, and then stand up again. Next, one child remains standing while the other bends his knees.

c. *Making waves with a sheet or blanket.* Move the sheet or blanket to make calm and stormy "waves"; the children can take turns, one at a time, to "dive" underneath the cloth. Then one child at a time lies down underneath it, and the other children move it around over her. In this way the child who is lying down can listen to "the sound of the sea."

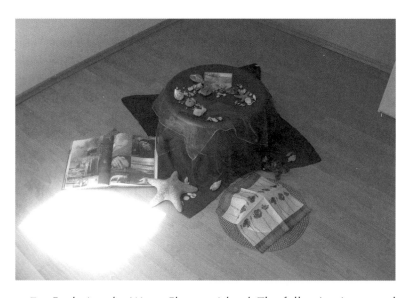

7. *Exploring the Water Element island.* The following items and foods were set up for the children to taste, touch, smell, and examine the Water Element with their senses: blue color scheme, a glass of water/salt water, bunch of celery, pulses (beans, lentils), sandalwood, seashells and singing bowls.

8. *Shiatsu.* The little turtles who want to be touched lie on their tummies in their sand nests (on their mats). The course leaders

crawl from one child to another and roll a balloon over the child's back, from the head, over the back, and down the legs, following the Bladder and Kidney meridians.

9. *Changing back into children.* All the turtles return to their sand nests (mats) and lie down under their blankets. The course leaders stroke each child (ask first), saying: "Now the turtle child turns back into the girl/boy XX [name of the child]." Then the child's head is uncovered. The child is asked to remain lying down until all the turtles have been changed back into children.

10. *Closing ritual.* The children form a circle. As a memento of this session, they receive a seashell for their treasure chest and a card with a picture of a sea turtle on one side and the three empowerment statements on the other. All together they speak the following empowerment sentences three times:

- I am calm.
- I trust myself.
- I trust life.

FIFTH WEEK: DESCRIBING THE FIRE ELEMENT— THE DRAGONS OF GOOD FORTUNE

1. *Entering into the Fire Element:*

   a. Everyone sits together in a circle around a Fire Element centerpiece. The children look and say what they recognize in the images. The centerpiece is composed of the following: red fabrics; a dragon soft toy; a clown; a magic wand; a colorful bunch of flowers; a lighted candle (be sure to take every precaution—e.g. use a glass lantern); postcards, your own photos, or pages from old calendars of a laughing face; pictures of fire; pictures of people who love one another kissing; pictures of bright landscapes full of flowers; pictures of boisterous children; and a picture of someone meditating.

   b. Supporting and guiding the discovery and exploration with the children, the group gives presence to the Fire

Element and gains access to the particular "place" that needs to be explored during the session.

2. *Describing the Kingdom of Smiles.*

Today we're going to visit the Kingdom of Smiles. The Kingdom of Smiles is a land of gorgeous colors. The fields are full of bright, sweet-smelling flowers, and there are colorful forests with trees where you can make a wish. There are lots of cheerfully colored houses throughout the land. In the middle of the kingdom, there's a wonderful big castle with gold turrets that sparkle in the sun. In the castle lives the King of Gladness, who rules over his people with great goodness and sincerity. In order to get into the Kingdom of Smiles, we're going to turn ourselves into dragons of good fortune.

3. *Transformation into the Fire Element power animal—dragons.* The children lie in their caves. The Dragon of Good Fortune is a late riser and only gets up when the sunbeams tickle him on the nose. (The course leader goes round and tickles each child.) "Atchoo!" The Dragon wakes up.

4. *Tuning-in exercise for the Fire Element.* All the children jump up from a squatting position and clap their hands several times. The children tramp and stamp round the room, being careful not to hurt anyone. They play at being fire-spitting Dragons of Good Fortune, and then each dragon finds a rock to land on and settle down on (the children sit down on their mats).

5. *Story reading:*

After the Dragons have woken up and polished their wings, they rise into the air and fly to the splendid castle with the gold turrets. The King of Gladness has sent a messenger to say that all the Dragons are to make their way to the castle. High up in the clouds, the Dragons can smell the overwhelming fragrance of the brightly colored flowers and hear the inhabitants laughing. Exhilarated by all the warmth and affection, the Dragons land in the castle courtyard. There the King of Gladness is already waiting for them: "A warm welcome to you, my Dragons of Good Fortune, protectors of my country. In a village in my country, there has been misfortune. The inhabitants there are living in darkness and without happiness. You, my Dragons of Good Fortune, have been chosen to bring light, joy, and happiness back to these inhabitants. But before you carry out this task, it's necessary to train you, for the power of darkness is mighty. And only the Dragons of Good Fortune who are pure in heart will return unharmed." The Dragons retire to prepare themselves. They practice making scary faces, they spit giant, blazing flames into the air, and they put armour on their wings to equip themselves for the fight against the darkness.

At nightfall the Dragons go into battle. They fight fearlessly and courageously all night long, and the following morning too. At midday, when the sun is at its highest, the Dragons have finally conquered the darkness, and joy, light, and happiness can return to the village. Exhausted but happy, the Dragons of Good Fortune fly back to the castle.

Full of joy, the King arranges a festival to celebrate victory over the darkness. The climax of the festival is honoring the Dragons of Good Fortune by awarding them the Order of the Dragon. Proud and content, the Dragons return to their caves.

6. *The experimental phase—exercises to strengthen the Fire Element:*

   a. *Make faces, flap hands, and polish wings.* The children sit in a circle on their mats and make faces. Then they flap their hands. To polish their wings, they bend their arms at the elbows, pull their shoulder blades together, and make circles with their arms. Then they raise their right arm, still bent at the elbow, behind their head, grip their right elbow with their left hand, and stretch the right elbow across to the left side. Then they change arms and repeat.

b. *Welcoming joy*. The children kneel on their mats, spread out their arms, and raise their arms slowly. Then they let their arms sink down in front so that their hands are resting on their lap.

c. *Protecting friends*. The children kneel on their mats, hold their arms out at their sides, and then bring their arms round in front and hug themselves.

d. *Gasho (showing gratitude to joy)*. The children kneel on their mats, lay one hand over the other on their tummy, and then raise their hands level with their heart. As they breathe out, the children lean forwards and touch the floor with the palms of their hands.

e. *Dance with red streamers*. Before the session, lots of brightly colored scarves are scattered over the floor, with garlands of flowers among them. Then they are covered with a big black cloth.

    This symbolizes the village where the misfortune has happened. Each child receives a long red streamer fastened to a pole. They all stand around the black cloth, facing outwards, and swirl the streamers around in front of their feet. Then the children turn round, and together swish their streamers, harder and harder, over the black cloth to drive away the darkness. To finish, all the Dragons together pull away the black cloth and dance with the colored scarves and garlands.

Note: You can use a roll of red crepe paper to make the streamers. Cut the crepe paper into strips 3–4 inches wide and about 3 feet long. Stick each strip to one end of a bamboo potting stick or a cardboard paper towel roll, which should be at least 2 feet long. (You can get bamboo potting sticks at a hardware shop or garden center.)

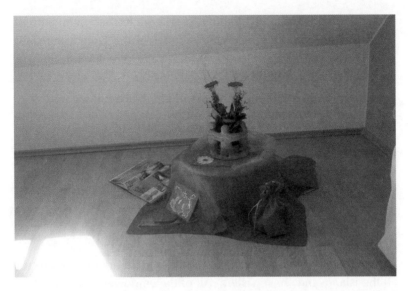

7. *Exploring the Fire Element island.* The following items and foods were set up for the children to touch, taste, smell, and examine the Fire Element with their senses: red color scheme; an orange; a red pepper; cocoa; a red candle; and rose essential oil.

8. *Shiatsu.* Treat the Heart/Small Intestine and Pericardium/Triple Heater meridians. The children lie down on their backs in a circle, with their heads towards the center; they then stretch out their arms to hold hands. All together, the children move their arms beyond their heads, so that their arms form the shape of a star. Beanbags are laid along their arms, and the course leaders crawl on all fours, with a relaxed body weight, over the beanbags on the children's arms.

9. *Changing back into children.* Each child is awarded the Order of the Dragon by the King of Gladness in the castle courtyard. For this, each child in turn has to step into the middle of the circle and stand in front of the King. After the awards ceremony, the Dragons fly away to the Land of Dragons. Each dragon goes back into its hole. To finish, the Dragons are transformed back into children.

10. *Closing ritual.* The children form a circle. As a memento of this session, they receive the Order of the Dragon for their treasure chests. (Photocopy the image of a friendly dragon on to red card and stick clear film over it. The chain for the Order can be made out of gift ribbon or yarn.)

All together, the children speak the following empowerment sentences three times:

• I am happy.

• I listen to my heart.

• I am a good friend.

Bringing the Course to an End

The children form another circle. In the middle are the pictures of all the islands they have visited. All of the empowerment sentences are repeated, and in turn the children are allowed to go once into the middle of the circle to get their treasure chest, which holds the symbols and empowerment cards for each Element.

For each child the course leader says: "XY—it's been lovely to have you with us! Goodbye, XY." All the children repeat: "Goodbye, XY."

A Community Five Element Event: A "Construction Site" That's Lots of Fun for Kids—An Outdoor Action Day

To conclude our series of examples, we would like to present one more, larger project. We conducted this event as an outdoor community and family activity day. The concept allows for numerous variations, whether at a school festival, a kindergarten activity, or on a smaller scale for an indoors or outdoors child's birthday party. The example can serve as an inspiration to show how the Five Elements can be experienced with simple, everyday materials.

The Community Event
The Movement Construction Site as an Experiential and Learning Concept

The Movement Construction Site represents a traditional Western pedagogical concept for movement training in kindergarten and sports instruction in primary school. The basic idea comes from educational theorist Klaus Fischer Miedzinski and has been used in various spheres of pedagogical practice for more than 15 years. The concept of the Movement Construction Site rests on the notion of employing readily available materials and objects to develop a wide range of movements in children of preschool and primary school age. This project gives us the possibility to support children's development through the stimulation of the nervous system with normal movement activities in the environment. The simple activities created allow children to have multiple levels of experiences with the intention of offering different qualities of stimulus for them to grow and learn. They work with everyday materials and tools with their hands and learn things about their own bodies as they come into contact with other children in a cooperative way. Even simple building materials (boards, beams, car tires, barrels, etc.) and ordinary objects (cardboard, carpet remnants, etc.) promote fantasy and ingenuity in children. Building and construction promote opportunities to experience planning with others in order to enable their movement and behavior to be similar to normal daily routines that are practical. Direct orders from the instructors and supervisors of the activities are discouraged as much as possible. A responsible measure of risk taking belongs in the Movement Construction Site and helps make it attractive and exciting for children.

In the following, we linked the idea of the Movement Construction Site with the Five Elements and the result was an exciting Five Element experience for adults and children.

The Movement Construction Site and the Five Elements

Our Movement Construction Site was held in Germany on a Saturday in July. Many hands pitched in to make it a success: colleagues and graduates of our institute, teachers in training, parents of children in our groups, and a variety of neighbors.

Our institute is located in a village with 1400 inhabitants. Nicely renovated half-timbered houses are characteristic of the village center, along with little cobblestone streets, which were closed off to traffic on this day. The residents of these cobbled alleys opened their romantic inner courtyards, and made them available for some of the activity stations created for the Movement Construction Site.

The first station or court, just after the roadblock, was called the Welcome Court.

Here we provided information leaflets about the Movement Construction Site. Five stations were created in correlation to the Five Elements and were indicated by the corresponding Element and its related color. A long piece of colored fabric was strung from a post at the entrance to each station. Upon visiting each station, the children were to cut off an inch of fabric to put in a kaleidoscope that they had made from a cardboard tube, so that at the last station they would have five scraps—one each of green, red, yellow, white, and blue inside. Although there were only five scraps, in the kaleidoscope there were suddenly an unexpected number of patterns and color combinations to be seen. This had a great fascination for the children. The kaleidoscope became a symbol of the Five Elements and their multiplicity and brightness.

The beginning of the village street was taken over by a huge labyrinth/maze—this was the Wood Element station. A mountain of moving boxes, large appliance boxes, and various obstacles formed the labyrinth. In the center of this maze stood a ladder covered in corrugated tubes. Once one had wandered through the labyrinth as far as the ladder, they could climb up high and see "the big picture" of what they just walked through.

The court for the Fire Element had a Native American motif. A great teepee with a cooking fire, straw mats on the ground, and bundles of straw for cushions invited visitors to linger around the fire. From old carpet tubes, drums of various sizes had been made and covered with "skins" from plastic sheeting. The group drumming and the wild Native Americans dancing around the fire—sometimes more, sometimes less—helped to build the "inner fires" of experience. With red faces, much enthusiasm, and just as much laughter, children and adults alike took part in the "fire and flame" activity.

In the next courtyard, the largest, the student teachers had set up all of the Elements simultaneously with activities that combined all of the Elements moving playfully in and out of each other. This station represented the Earth Element, as it symbolizes the transition and interaction of all of the Elements. In the center of the court, the classic Movement Construction Site was ready with materials for building and constructing (Wood Element): boards, wooden chests, car tires, bales of straw, ropes, round beams, drainpipes, and small balls. Here, the children could climb, balance, build, dismantle, and experiment according to their imagination, age, and abilities. To gather experiences with the Fire and Earth Elements, children could prepare flatbread by themselves. There was flour to be ground with a stone, dough to be kneaded, and flatbreads to be formed and baked on an open fire. At another station (Earth Element), there were piles of red, yellow, and black sand, as well as various sizes of gravel to play in. Another area had a self-made cable car which was very popular and brought lots of joy (Fire Element). The ride ended in a heap of straw. There were giant soap bubbles to blow with the help of rings made from coathangers, which everyone watched in amazement as they hovered in and out of all the activities (Metal Element). A water slide, like a slip and slide, which was made slippery with soap and ran flat across the ground, was also a favorite. With much enthusiasm and interaction with each other, the children tried out various body positions while sliding. A washtub filled with water offered the chance to make various objects sink, bob up and down, and float. Small self-made wooden boats, powered by balloons, flitted across the water (Water Element).

The next stop on the way was the Earth Element court/station which, like the Wood station, was set up on the old village alley. Here, large old tubs were set up filled with earth, and hidden treasures were planted to be dug up. We got soil from a construction site, mixed it with sand and water, and scattered various semi-precious stones of different shapes and colors throughout the dirt (inexpensive tumbled glass beads, mermaid tears, marbles, collected rocks, and slate pieces that were smooth). The children had to dig with the full length of their arms to find the treasures. After some initial skepticism, the adults too began to dig into the dirt—and had lots of fun as well! To shorten the waiting time, others could paint with earth colors near the tubs. These colors were made up from various soils, and vibrant color pictures resulted. Everyone who visited the Earth station was immediately recognizable by the spattering of mud on clothes, faces, and hair.

After this station, the path led to the next court, where the Metal Element was the theme. A wooden rectangular frame, 9 × 18 feet, made from posts hammered into the lawn and roofing slats, awaited the children and adults. Large brightly colored bundles of ribbons and yarn could be threaded in the multidimensional frame to form a giant spider's web. Everyone got so involved that by the end not just the frame but the whole courtyard was spun into a web. Now it was time to try to cross the web, in every possible way. "Will I get through here?" To make this event still more colorful, children could have their faces painted with the spider's web, or they could make truly gruesome tickle-spiders from thick pipe cleaners.

Beside the giant spider's nest, there was a balloon room for a "contact bath." The small room was half filled with balloons, with a net before the doorway to keep the balloons inside.

One more courtyard invited everyone to experience the Water Element. Everything was done up in shades of blue. The walls were covered with pictures of fishes and marine animals painted by the children, and a home-made murmuring spring and hanging waterworks rounded out this station. There was also a wading pool with various tubes and containers available for experimenting. But the big hit was the water tarpaulin (a large water-resistant tarp): two or three children or adults would lie next to each other on a mattress. Several helpers would then let down over them a plastic sheet of blue-colored water, sometimes flapping it and sometimes touching them directly; or sometimes they would simply enjoy the color of the light through the water. Mostly everyone had goose bumps or a tingling in the stomach, wondering: "Will the sheet hold, or will I be taking a shower in a moment?"

The Movement Construction Site concluded with a quiet space. Here, one could paint, listen to quiet music, rock in the hammock, or listen to stories being read aloud. And, of course, there was a refreshment court at hand, where food and drink were available at any time.

In the beginning for us was the question: which age group did our activities appeal to the most? The action day was created for the whole family, and in fact, large and small took part in everything. We watched with interest when, for example, a group of 13-year-old boys ran swiftly through the alley with raucous shouts, and yet, at the end of the day, it was these same boys who, covered in mud and paint, were the last to leave and make their way home. This, then, was our own experience. After some hesitation and tentativeness, all age groups took up the offer of many of the stations, and we observed the adults participating as fully as the children. Many asked with hope that a similar event could be held the following year.

For us, as the initiators, we were especially pleased to learn, in the days after, that some of our suggestions could be found in home gardens—whether it was a spider's web in smaller format using strips of old clothes, or the home-made cable car with parts from the mountaineering store. And there were criticisms, too, since some of the mud spots wouldn't come out in the wash. But, for us, the goal had been achieved, namely that of offering suggestions that were of interest to all age groups and could be applied by children and parents together in their own homes.

Resources

Books

Kalbantner-Wernicke, K. (2010) *Shiatsu für Babys und Kleinkinder.* Energetische Entwicklung, Förderung und Behandlung. München: Elsevier.

Kalbantner-Wernicke, K. and Haase, T. (2012) *Baby Shiatsu: Gentle Touch to Help your Baby Thrive.* London: Singing Dragon.

Kalbantner-Wernicke, K. and Wernicke, T. (2011/2014) *Samurai-Shiatsu. Mit Shiatsu fit für die Schule.* München: Kiener.

Kalbantner-Wernicke, K., Wernicke, T., and Wray-Fears, B.J. (1998) *Die Fünf Elemente im Leben von Kindern.* München: Kösel.

Wernicke, T. (2014) *Shōnishin: The Art of Non-Invasive Paediatric Acupuncture.* London: Singing Dragon.

Websites

www.aceki.de: aceki e.V., Academy for Child Development, Alte Dorfgasse 13 65239 Hochheim–Massenheim.

www.baksev.de: German Association for Infant and Child Shiatsu Therapists.

www.kookoundfreunde.de: Samurai Community Projects, Karin Kalbantner-Wernicke, Alte Dorfgasse 13 65239 Hochheim.

www.shiatsumassageinstitute.com: Shiatsu Massage Institute, USA.

www.shonishin.de: Japanese Children Acupuncture.

www.whywaldorfworks.org: The Association of Waldorf Schools of North America (AWSNA).

About the Authors

Karin Kalbantner-Wernicke is a Shiatsu Instructor and Physiotherapist with qualifications in pediatric physiotherapy (Vojta, Bobath), sensory integration, and psychomotoric therapy. She is a founding member of the German Shiatsu Society as well as of the Federal Association for Baby/Children Shiatsu Practitioners. With 30 years of experience in teaching, Karin now focuses on instructing certification classes for Baby/Children Shiatsu in Germany, Austria, Switzerland, Great Britain, Hungary, the Netherlands, Spain, Japan, and the United States.

Thomas Wernicke, MD, MA, is a Licensed General Practitioner with qualifications in complementary medicine and Chinese and Japanese acupuncture, as well as manual therapies including craniosacral therapy and osteopathy for adults, children and babies, psychosomatic therapy, and homeopathy. He is the Medical Director of the Therapeuticum Rhein-Main.

As a member of the Japanese Scientific Society for Shōnishin, he is Training Manager for Daishi Hari Shōnishin in Europe.

Karin and Thomas are founders of the therapy center Zentrum for Therapeuticum Rhein-Main and the training center aceki e.V. As well as teaching, their main concern is research about children's development from the Eastern and Western points of view. They are sought-after lecturers on this topic, and numerous scientific articles have been published by them in many countries, including Japan. Both are founding members of the International Society for Traditional Japanese Medicine. They live in Hochheim, Germany.

Bettye Jo Wray-Fears, MA, LMHC, LMT, is a Licensed Mental Health Counselor and Shiatsu Therapist/Instructor. Bettye Jo completed her Shiatsu Practitioner Certification with Karin and trained in the Five Elements with the Traditional Acupuncture Institute SOPHIA Program. She has dedicated her continued studies and therapeutic practices to integrate Eastern and Western approaches to human development for children, individuals, parents, and families. With a background in Buddhist philosophy, Eastern medicine, and modern and traditional psychological approaches, Bettye Jo offers psycho-education therapy to all ages, incorporating body–mind–soul approaches to support growth and self-awareness for balanced living. She is the founder of the Shiatsu Massage Institute, as well as the Energetic Development Institute, where classes and trainings in the Five Elements, Baby/Children Shiatsu, and other life-span developmental approaches are offered. Bettye Jo continues to teach the Five Elements with Karin in Germany in the aceki e.V. certification programs.

Index